When the Voiceless Sing

When the Voiceless Sing

Love stories from our hero Caregivers

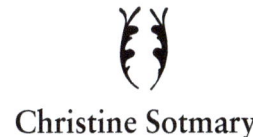

Christine Sotmary

What our readers think:
"*When the Voiceless Sing* opened my eyes to the power and rewards of the Caregiving experience. Instead of thinking about caring for a patient as a task, I now see it as mutual relationship with potential for the Caregiver's growth as well as giving support for someone who is vulnerable."
— Pat. W. New York City educator

"During our two year book club, using the manuscript for *When the Voiceless Sing*, we received very practical information from our discussions and are richer to know about dementia and the many issues involved in Caregiving. The book was down to earth, honest, and to the point and very useful in helping us be better Caregivers. We are grateful to be able to share these gifts in caring for our sisters and the people we meet each and every day."
— Sr. Patricia Burke from Graymoor Convent

This book is dedicated to a time when each and every Caregiver will get to tell their story to a world that is listening closely.

When The Voiceless Sing

Christine Sotmary, M.S., LAc., CPC

Published by:
Christine Sotmary, M.S., LAc., CPC
P.O. Box 513
Crompond, NY 10517
©2012 by Christine Sotmary

Sacred Life Publishers™
www.sacredlife.com
Printed in United States of America

All rights reserved. No part of this book may be reproduced or transmitted in any form or by any current or future means electronic or mechanical, including photocopying, recording, or by any information storage and retrieval system without written permission from the author, except for the inclusion of brief quotations in a review.

ISBN-13: 978-1477419427
ISBN-10: 147741942X
Library of Congress Control Number: 2012950138

Book Design: Loretta Reilly Design, Inc

Disclaimer
This book is designed to provide information about the subject matter covered. Any advice given in this book is soley the opinion of the author, based on the author's own experience. This book is sold with the understanding that neither the author nor the publisher is engaged in rendering medical, legal, psycholgical, financial, or any other professional services. If expert assistance is required, the services of a competent professional should be sought.

Every effort has been made to make the information in this book as complete and accurate as possible. The information is not guaranteed or warranted to produce any particular results. There may be mistakes, both typographical and in content.

Therefore, this book should be used only as a general guide.
The purpose of this book is to inform and entertain. Neither the author nor the publisher shall have liability or responsibility to any person or entity with respect to any loss or damage caued, or alleged to be caused, directly or indirectly, by the information contained herein.

> "Through caring for certain others, by serving them through caring, a man lives the meaning of his own life."
> — From *On Caring* by Milton Mayeroff 1971

These wise words were the jumping off point for **When the Voiceless Sing** which takes a close look at the trials and rewards of Caregiving. Caregivers are a special set of people who by choice or chance devote much of their own lives to the needs of others whether for just minutes a day, or as a full-time commitment to the exclusion of almost all other human interaction. By asking 22 Caregivers about their experiences **When the Voiceless Sing** gives voice to the daily challenges Caregivers face, how they find humor and sustenance in seemingly impossible situations, and how they have been able to manage their frustrations.

Would we find the courage, the love, the commitment, the skills and the support to take on this incredible role of Caregiver? The reader will come away with a much clearer understanding of what goes on behind closed doors when illness, special needs, disabilities and the demands of aging become the family's focus. They will also see how neighbors and friends step in when called upon and we get to ask ourselves what we would do in their place.

Contents

Dedication 5

Introductory thoughts by Stephen and Ondrea Levine 10

Acknowledgement 11

Preface 12

Section A: Caring as a way to help another flourish 15
Chapter 1: Fostering trust and growth in another 17
Chapter 2: Separate and together 27
Chapter 3: Devotion 35

Section B: What elements go into caring 43
Chapter 4: Knowing another 45
Chapter 5: Learning what comes of our caring and tweaking, always tweaking 55
Chapter 6: Rhythm of switching back and forth from the big picture to the individual moment 61
Chapter 7: Patience in caring 67
Chapter 8: Seeing us both honestly 75
Chapter 9: The courage of trust 83
Chapter 10: The humility in learning 89
Chapter 11: Building on our strengths and recognizing our weaknesses 95
Chapter 12: Hope for the present and possibilities for the future 101
Chapter 13: The challenge of the unknown 107

Section C: What is there to learn in caring 113
Chapter 14: Selflessness, loss of self and selfishness 115
Chapter 15: Having goals while living in the moment 123
Chapter 16: Can I care and can the other be cared for 129
Chapter 17: The commitment of caring 135
Chapter 18: Guilt and neglect 139
Chapter 19: Mutual or one-sided care for the long or the short of it 145
Chapter 20: Limits and boundaries of caring 151

Section D: Focus on caring for people 159
Chapter 21: Being connected by our caring for others 161
Chapter 22: Caring for myself 171

Section E: What caring does to organize our lives and give us meaning 179
Chapter 23: Caring organizes our life and our priorities 181
Chapter 24: The music of caring - themes harmony and flow 189
Chapter 25: The feeling of being "in place" or "at home" in our world 197
Chapter 26: Significant others 205
Chapter 27: Finding meaning in a life well-lived 211

Section F: What describes a life built around caring 219
Chapter a: Basic certainty 221
Chapter b: Living life is enough 227
Chapter c: Understanding and wonder 235
Chapter d: Autonomy through dependence 245
Chapter e: Caring in faith and belief 255
Chapter f: Caring as gratitude 263

Who are our hero Caregivers? 269
22 short biographies

About the Author 274

Resources 275

End Notes 276

Index of Caregivers 277

Caregiver Notes 278

Order Form 280

Introductory thoughts

by Stephen and Ondrea Levine

We care for hearts as they move towards the end of worldly relationships. We are blessed to be included at the bedside with the dying. Each experience breaks our heart and builds our strength. With that strength we are able to serve the dying and their Caregivers again and again.

We can be there not only for those who are in the last phase of their lives but also for their Caregivers because they are entering a new phase of their own. Each one is suffering a grief as do we all. We have never met anyone who was totally without grief. We let our grief sink from our mind into our heart so that we may heart to heart serve another.

This is the work on ourselves we were born to do. The healing we took birth for. It is the hardest and most wonderful work we will ever do. We are the worn and the blessed. It feels that we are half way between heaven and hell in so many ways. We end up taking responsibility for the life that was given us by aiding those whose lives are fleeting.
—*A message from our hearts... all the best, Stephen & Ondrea*

For more inspiring thoughts look for their book *The Healing I Took Birth For* by Ondrea and Stephen Levine

For other writings, videos and teachings from Stephen and Ondrea go to: http://levinetalks.com/

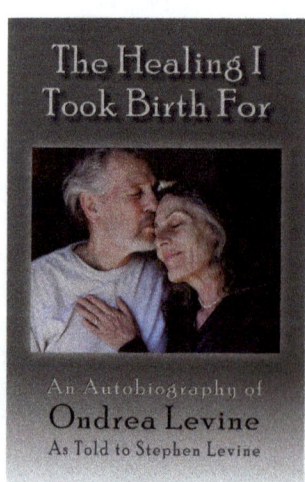

Acknowledgement

I want to especially thank all the Caregivers who took their time to be interviewed for this book. You can't see it on the page but as each question was answered from their full hearts there were tears and also smiles for special memories. I am thankful for the courage it took for these Caregivers to return to sometimes painful places of loss and grief.

I also want to thank the nuns at Graymoor Convent for our wonderful book club. Every month we would visit a different chapter of **When the Voiceless Sing** and reflect on our own experiences with Caregiving. It was my pleasure to witness them caring for each other during times of physical and emotional pain especially during times of loss for their close knit community.

I am grateful to Pat Walter, Lucy Gilbert, Elaine Strum and Libbie Rice for their generous comments.

And lastly but never leastly, I want to thank Joe Perez for being my muse and angel during this process. There would be no book without him and I am truly grateful for all his support!

Preface

Two years ago, in the middle of a Nor'easter rainstorm, I was doing some cleaning up in my tiny New York City apartment. On that fateful afternoon I made an amazing discovery. It appeared in the form of a tiny book that was hidden under many years of old tax returns and miscellaneous papers.

This little book was written by the philosopher Milton Mayeroff, and it was called *On Caring*. I had never seen the book before and had to assume that it had belonged to my husband Alan. Alan had died the year before, and this was the last file cabinet of his that needed sorting.

The book caught my eye for several reasons. I was amazed that someone could write an entire book about the singular topic of caring. I had been at my husband's side for eight years as his Caregiver during his journey with Alzheimer's. I had written a book about our experience together but I hadn't thought of looking at our lives through the singular lens of caring. I was curious about how Mayeroff could have so much to say.

The experience of being a Caregiver has inspired me to help others going through a similar experience. I have become the provider of a number of programs for family members who are Caregivers throughout Westchester County, a suburban area just north of New York City.

Through my own experience and now working with a wide range of Caregivers, I've learned that the role of Caregiving is multifaceted and more complex than most folks imagine. And when I considered that there is usually an emotional attachment involved with Caregiving, I realized there was much more I had to learn about caring. I had a strong suspicion that reading a philosopher's wisdom about its nature would be enlightening, not only for me, but for so many others who have had—and still are having—experiences as Caregivers. I was right; his observations were forceful and inspiring.

As the winds blew and the rains poured down that day, I read *On Caring* from cover to cover. I discovered that Mayeroff had understood much about the complex landscape of caring; more importantly perhaps, he had used a rich language to describe and expand upon it, allowing others to easily understand and more completely learn about their role as Caregiver.

Playing with these ideas made me think about writing this book: what if I put some of Mayeroff's ideas into the context of Caregiving and, based on my experience, started a dialog with Caregivers? What would they tell me? Could we begin together to create our own language to describe what we all are experiencing? How could we share this new language with others? How would I integrate my own experiences and expertise into this Mayeroff-inspired language?

Being a philosopher, he needed to describe what caring is and what it is not in dialectical terms. This boils down simply to everyday notions of opposites like the concept of yin and yang: you need hot to define what cold is not, for example, and you need black to define what white is not. From this premise, everything he said made sense. We will see more about the dialectic of Caregiving in Chapter 1.

So much of what Mayeroff was saying could be applied in caring relationships of all types and would especially help to make it easier for the Caregiver and those they are caring for - if the Caregivers only had the right tools!

While Caregiving has always been a part of our existence in society, there hasn't been much written about this intimate experience beyond the many "How to survive Caregiving" manifestos. We Family Caregivers take on the responsibility and don't much discuss the full range of what we are experiencing. Additionally, there is no formal training for the role, and when we get stuck it's been up to us to muddle through.

Whenever I ask Caregivers what they say when their family and friends ask how they are doing, I always get the same answer. They say they're fine and that ends the conversation. They rarely accept offers of help from others, not knowing what kind of help they might need or not wanting to be a bother to others.

Armed with this new language Caregivers could talk to each other, they could talk to their families and they could talk to their communities. They could ask for things that they previously weren't aware they needed. They could describe more accurately the experiences they were having, and identify problems--obvious and underlying--and then be given the comfort and support they so richly deserve.

The thought of creating the Language of Caregiving gave me the title of this book, *When the Voiceless Sing*. Song lyrics involve language. Until now, Caregivers haven't been given a place to sing, and oftentimes they haven't known the words to their song. I imagined that helping Caregivers discover that voice would help them find common cause with each other and the space to share experiences, laugh at absurdities, and support each other through the rough spots.

As you read, you'll quickly see that *When the Voiceless Sing* is not just a rehashing of Mayeroff's ideas, but a manifesto for growth for us all, as well as a practical guide through the tangle of situations and emotions encountered in Caregiving.

To stimulate the conversation, I have turned to the stories of 22 Caregivers, including my own, told within a loose framework constructed around Milton Mayeroff's observations. His original work spoke of all kinds of caring, for one's work, hobbies, art and relationships. For *When the Voiceless Sing*, I limited my questions for the most part to the caring for the people in our lives and work, to caring for ourselves and primarily to the role of being a Caregiver.

The 22 people interviewed either are now or had been Caregivers for someone who was frail, sick, disabled or dying. Some had had multiple experiences of Caregiving. I discovered that there does seem to be a personality that is attracted to Caregiving. I say this because I heard very little complaining from these Caregivers, not because they found the role easy but more importantly because they found it so fulfilling and meaningful. Not one regretted the experience. Of course there is the element of who would choose to tell their story. The more positive the Caregiving experience was the more likely a Caregiver might step forward to share theirs. Perhaps the book that explores what it means to reject the role of Caregiver when one is either first called upon or during the process is yet to be written. That certainly must be a difficult decision both to make and to live with.

The people I spoke with showed that they were willing to go above and beyond the expected, normal attentions, to bring comfort and dignity to the person they were caring for. Several were happy to have repeated the experience with more than one person in their life when they were called upon. I found this true in my own life as well.

I asked questions seeking to spark a memory and a story. They were not intended to narrowly channel the discourse, and many of the Caregivers wandered from the original question during our interview. I enjoyed the stories, no matter how far afield they wandered since we were looking for a language of caring and I had asked these Caregivers to speak freely. My instinct told me to leave the interviews intact for the most part. At the same time in the process of editing I have made any stories or story excerpts that I cut out from these pages available on the blog www.whenthevoicelesssing.blogspot.com so you can follow your favorite Caregivers and learn more about them.

I took stories from two Caregivers for each topic. Sometimes their stories are in back to back chapters but more often we return to each person in later chapters. Near the end of the book I've included a brief biography of each Caregiver's situation, whom they cared for and what their involvement was, so the reader can flip back and refresh their memory.

I made a point to interview people who were caring for others in a variety of situations. I interviewed therapists, teachers, business owners, project managers and personal trainers. I interviewed young and old, male and female, rich and poor, gay and straight. I interviewed people Caregiving for those who'd had strokes, multiple sclerosis, cancer, dementia, mental illness, autism, drug addiction, PTSD and more. I interviewed Caregivers who came from big families with a lot of support and those that had no one but themselves to carry this tremendous responsibility.

As we develop a deep awareness of what the Caregiving experience means to all of us and develop a language around caring to describe this experience the future explodes with possibilities. Fortified with this awareness and this language Caregivers will also be better able to express their own needs, share resources and ask for what will make their lives easier. Caregiver advocates and activists will be better equipped to discuss how to help Caregivers and put effective programs in place. Communities will understand that we all benefit when we care for our Caregivers.

Section A

Caring as a way to help another flourish

Chapter 1

Fostering trust and growth in another as we care

Author's reflections:
As we begin our journey with our Caregivers into their day to day world of Caregiving, we'll take a close look at what Caregiving is as well as what it is not. As we listen to the many stories that our Caregivers tell, three themes become important; Love, Caring and Caregiving. These words are not used interchangeably in this book. They have some slightly new meanings for our purposes.

Love, for the purpose of this book, is a feeling. It remains a feeling until it is acted upon. We can love people we haven't seen in years and never pick up the phone to call or visit. We can love people in faraway places but have no interaction in their day to day lives.

Caring is a much broader topic and can apply to many situations. As we take an active role in the lives of others we are caring for our families, friends, students, employees, relatives and our communities. There are many examples of caring later in this book.

In the most basic sense Caregivers are those who are called upon to provide a number of services and tasks for someone who is ill, frail or in some way vulnerable. They take time away from their own lives, dreams and goals to attend to another.

Musings on Mayeroff:
In caring, we see the potential in others and honor their need to grow by following their lead. We also understand what they need from us to help them grow.[1]

Author's reflections:
Caring is more than a simple feeling of loving someone. Neither is it simply a matter of acting as their custodian or keeping them safe. It begins with a dynamic interaction between two people; the ultimate goals for them both, whether understood or not, are personal growth and development.

There are various ways to achieve this. Seeing someone that I am caring for nourished and reaching their potential because of my care is how I personally grow and learn. I am constantly making sure that my caring is truly serving the other person. When it is not I change my approach.

In a friendship this caring can go back and forth with either person doing more of the caring from time to time. Regardless, both people still grow from the relationship. The ultimate way we know that our caring is working well is when the person we are caring for turns around and cares for others while still nurturing their own growth.

How do you nurture the person you are caring for's growth?

Debbie talks about helping her mother move into town

When my mother got into financial trouble and couldn't pay her mortgage we had to step in. My two sisters and I helped her sell our childhood house and move to a rental house in town.

Before this happened I had worked at the Maryknoll Seminary with their elders, so I tried to step back and see my mother in a similar way without putting my "daughter glasses" on. I would pretend to be an unrelated observer looking in and ask what was I really seeing? I needed to understand what she really needed and not just go along with what she was saying she wanted.

She seemed very happy once she moved to the rental home because it was much less of a burden. It was a cute little house and she had help with the lawn. Even though she had been attached to our childhood house she was actually miserable there. Things were falling apart and my brother-in-law couldn't keep up with it. He had a job and when she called him he couldn't come right over. This upset her.

Once she moved she really seemed happy because she didn't have to worry anymore. This decision to have her move was our way of nurturing her under the circumstances. Now my sister and her husband were literally around the corner and she was right in the center of town so she could walk, visit with friends and even walk to her part time job at City Hall.

Since her previous job was at the Town Hall she knew everyone in town and they could now come to check on her. In terms of finding her some work once the town had converted to computers they had to tell my mother that she couldn't work there full time anymore. When she moved into town they were good enough to find some part time work for her so she could earn a little money and feel good about herself. How many towns would do that? Not many! Most would say "You are old, get out." The fact that we helped her to move into town made all of this possible for our mother and it was great to see her blossom again.

When she suddenly passed away everyone came out to offer support. This was especially important because they also helped us to find homes for her seven cats!

Kellie talks about nurturing her dad's growth

Despite his Multiple Sclerosis it was easy to nurture my dad. I knew the things that he liked to do and that he was still able to do, like lecturing and writing. He communicated with scholars and publishers. He was quite happy then.

When he was first diagnosed he was upset that he couldn't do all the physical things he had done before, like playing hockey. Over time he had a change in his mindset and found things that he liked to do to replace what he had lost. It was almost like he grew into a new person.

I was able to nurture him by setting the ball in motion. I got him a computer. He didn't know anything about email or computers. That was twelve years ago and it was still early for knowing about these things.

At first we shared the computer but I decided he really needed his own so I gave it to him. The book that he wrote was a direct result of his having these new tools that I had provided for him. It was very rewarding for me to know I had helped him in this way.

Earlier in his life he had given lectures about economy in Africa but then he stopped when he settled down to become a local judge and raise a family. Because he was looking for ways to be less physical he realized that he could now start giving his lectures again. It was great that he could return to his lecturing because he was so smart in history and economics. He was able to walk with a cane once we brought him to the place where he would be lecturing. He couldn't drive because his feet were too weak. By helping him with transportation we were nurturing his growth as a vital man who was important in his field.

He was a great speaker, the best orator ever in my opinion! There was never a note—he could speak off the top of his head. The fact that he could get back to that ability was amazing to watch. My being able to nurture his growth came out of providing him with the computer and transporting him to the lectures. It would have been impossible for him to accomplish so much on his own. I was proud to be there for him.

He tended towards depression and had he not had all these outlets it's pretty certain that he would have suffered emotionally. At the time I was doing all this for my dad I didn't really think about it. Now looking back, he may very well have gotten depressed had he not had these gifts and my support.

He was able to stay active until my stepmom died. He died exactly a month after her, probably from a broken heart. You don't usually die of MS directly, maybe from the complications.

In thinking that I was nurturing him I concluded that he needed some rest after his loss because he seemed tired to me. Instead of the rest reviving him he got really depressed. He went downhill really fast and ended up in the hospital soon after and died within a few days. I wonder if I did the right thing or if I should have distracted him more.

Kellie talks about nurturing her step-mom during her vulnerability

During her earlier life my step-mother would never have let us see her in a bad way. She always needed to be in control. The emotional blossoming and trust came at the very end of her life. She finally needed to give up that control and let us help her.

During the later stages of my step-mother's cancer, allowing me to clean and change the feeding tube for her was a breakthrough. Before this she needed to control everything and everybody. She didn't want to seem vulnerable or have any help from us.

The way I gave her support allowed her to still maintain her dignity as she was giving up her control. I felt it was right to change her feeding tube instead of handing this over to strangers. This came out of my feeling close to her because I was her stepdaughter and also not wanting her to feel embarrassed. It was also symbolically showing my appreciation that she had fed me for many years.

Later she was also allowing us to see her as vulnerable when she finally let hospice come to the house. Once she was in hospice and not doing well I was there every day. My stepbrother was only able to get there once a week. By this time I think she took my presence for granted. When he would finally show up each week she would make a big fuss over him. I understood the situation.

In the end she really appreciated that I was there and I think her heart softened. At the end of her life she had gotten up to go to the bathroom and I was helping her and she just died right there in my arms. She was home when it happened and sometimes I stay over in that room because it feels very peaceful to me.

Author's reflections:
Once the Caregiving relationship is established, a subtle and unspoken feeling of trust often begins to develop. The care recipient grows to trust that the Caregiver will be there and do whatever is needed.

Caregivers rarely identify this feeling, that they have unwittingly encouraged to grow in the person they are caring for, as trust, or even recognize how profound it is. To know that someone understands that we will be there when they are at their most vulnerable needs to be celebrated. That we are counted on in often challenging situations is a testament to who we are as Caregivers.

Does the person you are caring for seem to trust you?

Debbie talks about trust with her mom

When my mother handed over her financial responsibilities to me and asked me to start making sure her bills were paid, she trusted me to take care of them. It was clear that she was overwhelmed and just needed to inquire about certain bills from time to time.

Trust is really a two way street in Caregiving. She trusted my sisters and me but it was hard for us to trust what she was saying. She would tell me and my two sisters different stories about her affairs or what was going on in her life. Her lack of being able to deal with a consistent reality was the main reason she got into so much financial trouble.

Since my sisters and I were in frequent contact with each other we finally realized what she was doing and realized we needed to step in. Right before she died she finally had started being a bit more dependable and we were just starting to be able to trust what she was telling us. This being better able to cope with reality might have happened because she was happier in her new situation.

Kellie talks about her grandfather's losing trust and becoming more assertive

I didn't feel like my Grandpa was blossoming as much as my parents had while I was caring for him. Later, towards the end, when the stroke had taken its toll he became more assertive as to what he did and didn't want. In the past it had been a matter of him giving over control to us because he trusted us but that changed in the nursing home. In this new situation he was truly out of control of certain aspects of his life. That's when he finally started making an effort to take back some of his control. I don't think he trusted the staff in the home the way he had his family.

When he could no longer speak or write he would get mad when he didn't want certain foods, for example. That was a positive thing to me, as I watched him rebel. Before, he was very Presbyterian, nothing was going to bother him. Now that he was expressing a more emotional side he actually yelled at the nurse. Even if it was partly delusional he was becoming more emotional and directive.

Once they called and said he refused his medications because he thought they were trying to poison him. This was a low point in his being able to trust them. I went over to the home to talk to him and explained that they were trying to help him. He told me the medicine made him feel bad. I said we would adjust it and find out what was wrong. It was scary for me to see him like that because this was nothing like how he had always been. I gradually got to grow and be able to handle his new ways of behaving. I suppose I was now trusting his changes were a sign of his growth and a good thing.

Kellie talks about trust in her Caregiving for her grandfather, father, and step mom

There was never a time that any of my relatives didn't trust me completely. I could make decisions for them and care for them without questions. I see other people who lock horns during these times, but I was very lucky. Maybe the fact that I was an only child made it easier.

We were a very small family and very close before all the medical issues started. They knew how they had raised me and knew who I was so that fostered trust as well. They never questioned anything.

It did put a lot of pressure on me. I worried whether I was making the right decisions. I wondered how someone could have so much trust in me. I don't have that much trust in myself even. It was really based on our relationship because I'm aware that they didn't have to trust me, they had a choice. It's pressure to be in this role but also an honor.

I've always been uncomfortable with praise. Even though it was clear that I was trusted I never wanted to have any attention because of it. My mother was the same way.

At my grandfather's wake everyone came up and talked about how I took such great care of him and my parents and what a great daughter I am. I couldn't handle it. That was the hardest part for me to hear all that acknowledgment. If I could trust that I had inspired others to care for their loved ones with the same devotion that I had, that's all I would really want.

Musings on Mayeroff:
When we are assisting another's growth it is not our agenda we are following. We allow their direction to guide us and determine our response.[2]

Author's reflections:
Caring involves quite a bit of acceptance and surrender to another person. It is only natural to feel that we know a better way, that we know what's right, that our experience is the only truth. When we truly care it becomes more about the other person, their rhythms, their agenda, and their path.

In Caregiving we suddenly find ourselves more deeply in the service of another. Their needs often come first and our work becomes a fulfillment of these needs. I often liken it to dancing with a partner; the Caregiver takes on the role of the follower, allowing the person they are caring for to lead. Both roles are necessary but the care recipient sets the choreography and leads the dance.

In your Caregiving who sets the agenda for how things will unfold with you and the person you are caring for? Does control or trust enter the decision making process?

Debbie talks about how her sister set the agenda with their mother

My older sister set the agenda and looked into what was really going on with my mom. Because my mom was telling each of us a different story about her finances with the house it was difficult to trust anything she was saying.

My mom would make requests for money and smaller things she wanted and we would go along with giving her some money. At the same time we began to take over the big picture decisions regarding the house. Due to our lack of trust in what she was telling us we started taking more of the control. None of us could afford to help her pay her mortgage. We knew that.

My sister dealt with the issues of the property that the house sat on. I dealt with the tenant in the back of the house. Initially, my mom would go in and talk to the people in the tax offices and the government officials. It became clear that she just wasn't grasping what they were telling her. My sister took over and did all that research.

Once we got to talk to the officials we realized they were telling a different version of the story then we had heard from our mom. We concluded that she was misunderstanding what they had said to her or maybe it was some kind of denial on her part.

We also eventually learned that our dad had handled most of the issues concerning the house before he died. If we had known that earlier we wouldn't have let things go for so long. We really trusted her when we should have been more on our guard. We had always thought that our parents were more equal in dealing with their finances but going through the records we realized it was mainly his responsibility. You would think that as a kid you would know more about your parents' relationship. What we learned surprised us.

Another of the reasons we thought my mother was on top of things was that earlier in her life she had worked for an accountant. She was his main secretary. We didn't realize that her accounting office skills didn't translate into being able to handle her own financial affairs.

Kellie talks about setting the agenda with her step mom, dad and grandfather

Because they trusted me, I pretty much set the agenda with my dad and grandfather. They were happy to hand me the control. It went back and forth with my stepmother until the last six months of her life. As they all eventually got weaker and more tired, I needed to do more of the planning and take over more control. They couldn't think about what was needed and passed it to me, sort of the way Scarlet O'Hara did with Melanie in the movie **Gone with the Wind**. It ultimately has made me a very organized person.

Musings on Mayeroff:
We also guide those in our care to take care of themselves and their lives.[3]

Author's reflections:
How we encourage others to care for themselves is one of the trickiest roles we take on as Caregivers. The amount of trust that is required as we allow them to choose their path is phenomenal.

Finding ways to motivate those we are caring for to also care of themselves is one of the highest art forms. Too much guidance and they rebel, not enough and they get side tracked. Fostering self-initiation and self-direction goes a long way towards keeping someone else's life on track.

How do you encourage the person you are caring for to care for themselves?

Debbie talks about her mom taking care of her adopted cats instead of herself

My mother didn't tell us how many cats she was caring for. When we asked how many cats she had adopted she would say three or four. After she died we found seven. When it came to adopting so many cats, we tried to explain to her that she would have more money if she had less cats to care for. She could have had all the money she needed to care for herself without the additional expense of so many cats. Meanwhile she was always broke and asking us for money.

She wasn't connecting the fact that the more animals she had meant more food and medical bills for the cats and less money for herself. We also wondered if she was starting to cross the line between caring for the animals and just exhibiting hoarding behaviors. We tried to explain it as something she could relate to like if she wasn't spending so much on her cats she could take senior trips like her friends and her sister were able to do. She never really made the connection between her difficulties with self-care and caring for so many cats.

She may have had problems understanding what we were saying or making certain connections. Dyslexia runs in our family, along with Attention Deficit Disorder so maybe our lecturing to her wasn't the best approach. She was also stressed out because she was moving to a new home and maybe it wasn't a great time to be trying to get her to take better care of herself.

Kellie talks about helping her grandfather to care for himself

One important way I encouraged my grandfather to take care of himself was to not move in with him when he had his stroke. I allowed him to stay by himself, and we figured out ways for people to come in at least once a day. Meals on wheels came and we taught him how to use the microwave. Actually this was an earlier time, before he went to the nursing home, that he also got to blossom personally, now that I think about it.

With his first small stroke (TIA), we only had to take the car away because I didn't want him driving anymore. But we could leave him alone in the house that he had lived in since 1946. He was comfortable there and had a routine. He had people from church and his friends coming in every day. On weekends my girlfriend took him out for dinner at the pizza place. He loved that. I called him twice a day. He took his own pills. This lasted until he had a major stroke and needed full time care.

Musings on Mayeroff:

To facilitate growth we help those we care for to also care for things, ideas and people. We encourage them to discover the areas that they will choose to focus their attention on.[4]

Author's reflections:
Finding one's passion in life is a mysterious process. Most people can't name the reason they got involved in the things that they care deeply about. Often it turns out to be a mentor, a teacher, a coach or a relative who shows the way. Someone who has complete faith in our abilities and nurtures our interests might light the path.

Doing this for another is challenging and at the same time rewarding. Being an inspiration for another person, or being a role model can propel someone else towards a lifelong ambition.

They say that children learn more from who we are than from who we are trying to make them be. Thus we must be attentive to how we nurture an-

Kellie's friend reading to her Grandfather.

other person's passions. Being involved in our own work or hobbies helps them see possibilities for themselves. Helping them question, explore, face challenges, create and solve problems lays a great foundation for them to discover what it is they will devote themselves to caring about.

How do you help the person you are caring for get excited about life?

Debbie talks about her mom's excitement about moving into town

We helped our mom get excited about moving into town. We knew that the rental house would brighten her future. We reminded her that she could visit with my sisters' kids and her great grand-children. We made sure she was seeing people in the town. My mom was very outgoing but now she could see folks she knew more because she was in town. My mom's lifelong friends would come and take her out. They would talk to her. She looked forward to their visits. She started becoming much happier and her mind was even getting clearer.

What I saw most was that she was more relaxed about things. Once she let go of the idea of keeping our childhood house and got over being embarrassed about the foreclosure she could relax.

She was excited about being in town. She became involved with the Board of Elections and also helped out at the youth center. Most of this was located at the Town Hall which was now just down the road from her rental place. I saw a big change in her once she was closer to the people and things that really meant something to her.

Kellie talks about helping her dad get excited about his work

I knew that my dad had a tendency to depression. I was able to give him a computer to use for reading, writing and communicating with others in his field of economics and history. I would talk to him about how he was helping other people even though he could no longer walk very far.

He was proud of being able to return to lecturing. He wrote a book on the history of slavery and the Underground Railroad on his new computer. From his earlier research he already knew a lot about Africa and was really into issues of equality and freedom.

Here he was a blond haired, blue-eyed guy who was very troubled by inequality! He helped a lot of people of color but due to his modesty he wouldn't admit to it in public. It is probably what kept him going.

Kellie talks about keeping her grandfather excited about baseball

My grandfather and I would talk about baseball. My husband listened to baseball games with him. My Grandpa could remember everything about baseball.

As a young man he was a pitcher who was scouted by the Brooklyn Dodgers. Unfortunately the war came and he enlisted instead of going to baseball camp that summer.

One time when my mom lived in Cooperstown and because she worked for the state, we got into a historic baseball place that you normally couldn't. There I met a guy who had been a pitcher for the Dodgers and a contemporary of my grandfather's. He actually remembered grandpa as the ambidextrous pitcher from a Monroe high school that they were trying to recruit. All the college aged guys were going off to war so the teams were showing up at the high schools to find players.

That day in Cooperstown this pitcher ended up writing my grandfather this amazing note. I gave it to my grandpa and he always kept it on him. He was such a humble person that he didn't think anyone would remember him, especially a Major League pitcher. He would get excited every time I mentioned his letter.

Chapter 2

Separate and together

Author's reflections:
Separateness is an aspect in a relationship that includes two separate people who are able to keep their personalities and individuality intact while both allowing the other to freely grow into their own potential. Togetherness is the aspect of these same two people joining together in a relationship either out of desire or need to help foster an environment that sponsors the maximum growth in the other.

When two people enter roles of the Caregiver and the person being cared for there arises a complicated dance with an ever changing landscape. Just as in a dance the partners need to feel comfortable with how close they are dancing, watching to not trip over each other's feet but remaining close enough to keep the connection in what they are creating. This isn't easy but when it is accomplished both partners benefit and grow.

We start with two possible situations from Milton Mayeroff that are pitfalls easily stumbled into, liable to take us away from this delicate balance of separate and together and the integrity and rewards of a truly caring relationship.[5]

The first occurs when a Caregiver choses an excessive togetherness without a mutual consent and sets the agenda for the other person—essentially, assuming the responsibility for their life—and puts themselves in the driver's seat, thereby robbing the person they are caring for of his/her independence and possibly their positive energy and motivation. Growth for both people is stifled, and the end result is unproductive and frustrating for both.

The second danger, which also involves excessive togetherness, is that the Caregiver becomes so taken up by the other's needs that they lose a clear sense of who they are and what their own needs are. This is a common occurrence and is referred to as Caregiver Syndrome. It's ultimately a lose-lose situation, because for a Caregiving relationship to be successful, a Caregiver must remain emotionally strong and separate in order to meet the others' needs: growth and fulfillment are not possible for either party when one gives oneself over completely to the caring for another. There needs to be a degree of separateness for things to go well.

Have you ever felt as if you were losing a clear sense of yourself in your Caregiving relationship? Why do you think this happens?

Terry talks about losing herself while caring for her dad

I did feel that I was losing myself when the situation with my dad got worse. This happened as things got more critical, like when I first found out about my dad's cancer and how serious it was. I needed to find out as much information as I could about who we should connect with and who was the best person to handle the situation in terms of medical advice and treatment. Did we need a second opinion, a third opinion? I sort of put everything else aside in my own life. I shut out everything else until I could be sure we were at the right place for him. Once I felt comfortable with the doctors and the situation then I could get some of my life back.

The next time I felt that I started to lose myself in the situation was when he started to spiral downward. An example was when my dad was told that he would be going into hospice. At that point I spiraled out of control emotionally because I knew what that step meant. At the same time it was important for me once he was settled in hospice to constantly monitor that he was comfortable. I again felt like I had to put my life aside because I wasn't sure I was doing everything I could and I started second guessing myself.

How I handled the being separate and together was to know that when I was with him it was "Dad time" and when I was at work it was "work time". It was hard but I had to set up those boundaries. I couldn't allow myself to get too distracted at work or my work would have suffered. I was lucky that there were four of us taking care of my Dad, my mom, my sister and my brother all helped. I took care of all the medical arrangements. It was manageable because I could delegate the things I needed to others in my family.

It was important that I had people there to delegate responsibilities to, and it was also important that I had a flexible work situation. I worked from home when I needed to and also kept crazy hours to fit my work around the visiting hours.

I maintained my social life in a limited way to help keep my sanity. I would see friends who had been through similar experiences and understood what I was experiencing so that helped. I also learned how to pick up the phone and ask for help from them. It was important that I had friends I could do that with.

Joe P. talks about keeping his own identity while caring for his dad

I kept myself intact while I took care of my elderly dad. It was hard when I would go to visit him in Florida because I had to fit into his world but when I was in my own home in New York it was easier to set boundaries. I have my friends and a full life so I was able to manage his care without giving up too much.

Musings on Mayeroff:
The person we care for is separate from us. We must recognize and respect their needs and their right to make their own decisions when they are able.[6]

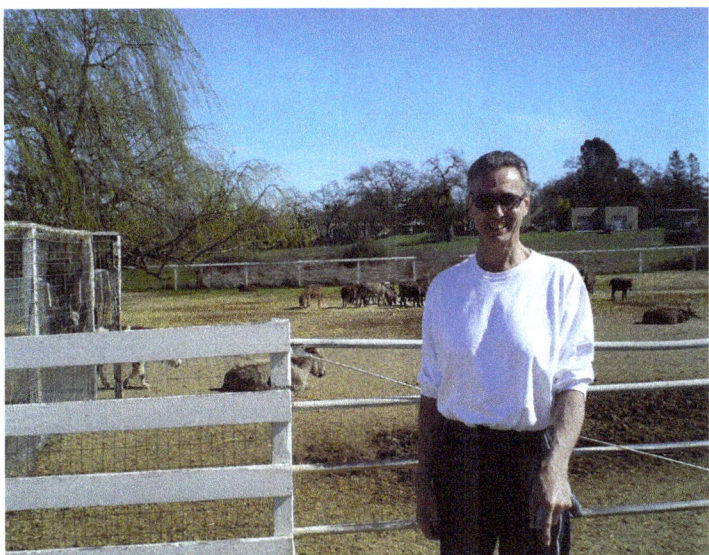

Joe P.

Author's reflections:
Respecting another person's dignity and understanding that they are still whole and functioning on many important levels allows them to have their own emotions and views without making them our own. This also allows us to respect the differences between us. In more limited ways this needs to occur even when someone is living with dementia, mental illness or other conditions that interfere with someone's personality.

On the other hand, being empathic, having the ability to understand, sympathize and experience someone else's sadness, depression or pain, or even anger, despondency, etc., without becoming defeated is another positive attribute for a Caregiver when striving to maintain the delicate dynamic of a Caregiving relationship.

Were you able to maintain separate identities and appreciate the differences between you and the person you were caring for?

Terry talks about keeping each of their identities with her friend

My friend and I were going through similar things at the same time with our dying parents. We stayed separate from each other and acted more as sounding boards for each other. If only one of us had been having difficulties maybe the other would have played a larger role in the other's life but the way it worked out we just couldn't. It turned out that the fact that we were going through similar experiences also allowed us to understand each other more deeply.

Terry talks about keeping her separate identity while looking out for her mom

I can feel like I am losing myself in the details of my mother's life. With all there is to check on it is difficult for me to maintain a separateness from her. It isn't so much about her failing health but more about switching roles, she as the child and me the adult. I have to keep reminding her to do things and check on what's been done.

Often she may forget to do something including make doctors' appointments. I don't have much patience with her. My sister can talk to her more calmly. My style is more businesslike and curt, "Where are the keys? Did you sign that paper?" etc. It actually might be more that that is my way of fighting to stay emotionally separate and not get lost in the situation.

Joe P. talks about the way he approached difference with his dad

I was myself and he was his self and somewhere along the line I realized it wouldn't serve any purpose if I became overwhelmed by his way of thinking or got lost in it. He needed someone to be more objective on the outside to help him accomplish things that he needed to get done.

He was scheduled to go to doctors to have certain things checked. He would set up the appointment and then cancel it because he didn't want to deal with their office situation at that time. He was not a patient person. He hated to sit in a doctor's office waiting to be called.

It became my job to get him to go to these appointments. Since I don't mind going to the doctor I had to really try to understand his feelings about not wanting to go. I didn't try to convince him that my way was right. I used the things I knew about him to try to convince him to take care of himself. That way his dignity could stay intact.

I approached him with logic and suggested if he didn't go now he would have to wait 3 months and that's a long time to wait if something is bothering you. I used the idea of not wasting this time to try to persuade him to do things he was reluctant to do. I also used logic to say he could also get seriously sick if he waited.

The thinking for me was to come up with ways for him to understand the necessity of not missing his appointments. This allowed him to solve his own problem and we could stay separate as complete people with our own histories and experiences. I am a strong problem solver so this is how I approached the situation.

Musings on Mayeroff:

We learn much about ourselves by following the growth and direction of another. We respect their integrity, their own sense of wholeness, and any direction we offer them is to further their growth.[7]

Author's reflections:
It is an act of great generosity to be supportive of another person's journey.

To carefully monitor what they need by watching their appreciation, even to see them exhibit snippets of sheer joy, and to change our own behavior to encourage these heartening behaviors is usually more difficult to accomplish than it sounds. At the same time, we learn much about our own values, strengths and relationships in the process.

What did you learn about yourself by attending to the person's you cared for need to flourish and maintain their dignity?

Terry learns about herself as a Caregiver by comparing herself to the lack of care that her great aunt was experiencing on her side of the family

Indirectly I learned a lesson about my commitment to my father's care and how I helped him maintain his dignity by being able to compare my care to a negative experience within my family.

My 90 year old great aunt in Florida has been having blood clots in her leg that have traveled to her lungs. She was in the ICU at the hospital. My mom and I travelled all the way down to Florida to visit her. We were anxious for my aunt to know we loved her and were worried about her. We wanted her to feel that she was important to us.

When we arrived at the hospital it surprised us that she was all alone in the room. She mentioned that her daughter had taken her family to Disneyland instead of staying with her to see what was going to happen with her health. My mother and I were shocked at this behavior. We saw that not everyone is as concerned as we are with the relationship they have with a loved one and their care. The idea of commitment and togetherness were missing in this situation.

On the way home I reflected on my great aunt's situation. I learned something about myself by looking at the situation with this part of my family. I had been able to take on the Caregiving responsibility with my Dad but not everyone has someone like me. I am proud that I could do that for him. I wish my other relatives were more like me and my mom and that my aunt had someone to help her feel supported and loved.

Terry talks about the difficulties of caring for her dad

What was difficult about caring for him was that my father and I never really got along. We were two separate people with similar characteristics. When we were drawn together because of his illness the walls never really came down between us. I could care for his health but not for his spirit and emotions. He kept himself very locked away and unavailable.

I resented the situation at first because my brother had always been the one that my father favored. I thought, "Let my brother do this," but he was incapable of it.

I was able to overcome my resentments and do what was needed to be done. Once I did take the controls I started to feel bad about the fact that my father and I hadn't gotten along and that I had had a difficult relationship with him. Sadly only after he died did I finally realize how intelligent he was as we were going through his things.

What made it hard for us to be close was that I'm very similar to him. I can talk to my friends and coworkers about anything but I can't talk to my family. I wish I wasn't like that. I'm not sure that he or I flourished or grew during the time I cared for him and I feel sad about that.

Terry talks about the difficulties of caring for her mother's growth

Maybe because of the burnout and stress from taking care of my dad I'm having trouble caring for my mother. What I've learned about myself is that I have even less patience now with my mother than I had with my dad. It's so hard. I try to feel the opposite, to be more generous, but I'm having less and less patience with her. I also resent that my brother who lives in the same building as her doesn't step up and handle things. Why am I the one who always has to do this? I can never catch a break.

What I'm learning about myself is that I'll have to learn how to get my brother, sister and mother to do more for themselves and set good boundaries. I have to learn that I can't be there every step of the way. I need to be more separate from them to renew myself and reflect on our relationships. Just being together and getting the job done isn't working for me or my mom. I don't see either of us flourishing the way things are now.

For my mother's self-respect she needs to learn independence. Recently she's been pretty good about picking up the checkbook and paying bills. It's a matter of letting her feel the pride when she can master these tasks. I am growing more separate as I encourage her to take on more responsibilities for herself. This has benefitted both of us.

Terry talks about her frustrations with the lack of her brother's growth

What is especially hard in a caring situation is not seeing any change or growth in the person you are caring for. My brother is getting worse. I can't depend on him to help with our mother and now he has his own health issues. I need to stay separate from his care so I can focus on our mom. He has his wife and I would only hurt the situation to be more involved with him. I'm too upset with him to even be rational.

He has completely shut down since my dad got sick and died. Plus he had his own surgery for cancer. He's depressed but he won't do anything about it. His wife cries to us about him.

I'll have to learn to only be a Caregiver for my mother and let go of everything else.

Joe P. talks about respecting his dad to foster his growth

I actually hadn't realized that I was such a good problem solver until my dad got older. I certainly had never dreamed as a younger man that I would ever be in this role with my dad or be good at it. I had always deferred to my dad because he was a powerful man who knew himself and what he wanted. I learned that I not only could problem solve when it came to caring for my dad but that I could present things in a way that was more palatable to him.

I grew and he grew from his being able to see me as a separate individual who could help him. He had previously only seen me as his child who would always be dependent on him. He didn't express the difference this made in his later life directly in words. Instead he did start to ask for my advice in his affairs, which was a new way for him to deal with me.

Musings on Mayeroff:
We need to evaluate our approach to how separate or together we have chosen to be to those we care for. We monitor the results of our actions through our observation of their reactions, moods and energy levels. We then evaluate these observations for how to modify our approach in the future.[8]

Author's reflections:
In Caregiving it is important to keep a close watch on those we care for by checking on the effects of our approach to a situation. This especially holds true when it comes to how close we can be before we might start to interfere with another's personal integrity while we are caring for them. What part do we play in the decisions they need to make? Are they flourishing under our care or becoming more apathetic?

To avoid burnout it is also important for us to know how separate we need to be to preserve our own individuality, to recharge our batteries and to maintain our health and wellbeing.

In science they call this process an outcome study. Researchers try out their hypotheses and see if they achieve positive outcomes for the participants in the studies. Once the results of the study are gathered they can be turned into recommendations for best practices so that the positive outcomes can be repeated.

As lay people, instead of observing, we more often wrongly assume that our approach will work. We forget to check on whether our expectations are actually born out. By carefully observing the results of our approach we can become alert to when we need to change and find a better way. This involves seeing ourselves and the person we are caring for as both separate as individuals and together as a team working for the benefit of both in this caring partnership.

Were you able to adjust your approach to a situation when things needed to change? Did you get more involved or less involved and why?

Terry talks about being able to adjust how involved with different family members she needs to be

I often change tactics on my job as a project manager so it was easy for me to adjust to his needs as I took care of my dad. I found this more with his health care than with his emotional wellbeing. As his health started to fail I was eventually able to adjust to his needing hospice and what my role would be as he lived out his final days.

Issues are more difficult for me when it comes to the rest of the family and needing to adjust. I'm learning that I'll just have to leave my brother out of my focus to better take care of my mom.

Joe P. speaks about adjusting as he cared for his dad

It wasn't hard for me to adjust because everything I did came from the place of loving my dad and the tremendous respect I had for him. I saw what his needs were and did the best I could do for him. As he needed more help I grew more involved and hired neighbors to help out. I would go visit more often and I started finding out more about his medical issues. Since I was in New York and he was in Florida I was able to maintain my own life at home in between caring for him. If I had been living with him things might have been different.

I didn't compare how he was as he became more frail to how he was as a younger man because I'm growing old too and these changes have to happen. I didn't judge him to be any less of a person as his body declined.

I found it a very exciting process to leave my mind open, to learn how to change my approach and when I was successful I would have fun with the experience.

Chapter 3

Devotion

Author's reflections:
Devotion is a state of being enthusiastically dedicated and loyal. It is the quality that turns love into caring and caring into Caregiving. It is an end product of time and effort. It is not something that happens overnight. It implies profound dedication, for our purposes of discussion, towards another person. Devotion rarely arises at the onset of caring, but it takes time to mature. For me, it is caring in its truest sense because it is an outgrowth of trust and knowing another person intimately.

To round out our thoughts on devotion, it is helpful to mention how devotion towards another person can go awry and, bringing back Milton Mayeroff's notions of the dialectic, we'll see what devotion is not. Neglect would be the polar opposite of devotion but there are many degrees of dedication between devotion and neglect. Caregivers are continually struggling with these notions and often feel guilty about not being devoted enough.

Importantly, says Mayeroff, devotion is incomplete if there is not a giving of one's whole self. This giving of one's self needs to be done in such a way that both partners benefit and grow. Despite the best intentions, people may be prevented from this total involvement based on their fears. Something is clearly holding them back, perhaps a fear of losing themselves in the caring. Those Caregivers who hold back often feel ambivalent about their caring.[9]

Musings on Mayeroff:
Devotion, or protracted, ongoing caring, is the substance and character of Caregiving. Being consistent during adversity and overcoming problems such as the declining health of the person we are caring for or facing our financial challenges are an expression of our purpose as a Caregiver; they free us to experience the merging of what we think we should do and what we are quite content to do. There is no need for us to hold back in our devotion because it is what fulfills us.[10]

Author's reflections:
Some Professional Caregivers feel they have been called to their work by spiritual or religious forces. Families, however, are usually surprised when they are called on to care for a frail or sickly member of their clan. Rarely has this huge responsibility been a part of one's game plan for life. When it does become a reality, however, the day-to-day running of peoples' lives becomes upended and financial assets are often drained.

When a family member is called on to be a Caregiver, he or she may discover caring to be the most meaningful work he or she has ever done. Being able to meet challenges, becoming more sensitive and responsive to the person we are caring for, and generally feeling content in our role are the hallmarks of a successful Caregiver. Being positively involved over a number of years in another's care has the potential to be fulfilling and add meaning to our lives in ways that we never could have anticipated.

Are you devoted to your Caregiving over the long haul, not knowing what your future holds?

Debbie talks about her devotion to her husband's brother and sister-in-law as they care for his aunt

When we got back from visiting my husband's aunt who has Alzheimer's we wondered how long my husband's brother and sister-in-law could handle her direct Caregiving. Our sister-in-law has her own severe health problems. She may end up in a wheelchair someday and my brother-in-law will have to decide who he will be able to care for–his wife or his mother.

In terms of the long haul, we are dedicated to helping them as much as we can even though we might not be the primary Caregivers taking care of my husband's aunt. We don't live nearby but we can visit more often and make sure they are OK. I've promised to call our sister-in-law more frequently and my husband will call his brother. I'll call in the morning when my sister-in-law is feeling better. She has shared personal things with me so I think it will help her to know that we are there. Since my brother-in-law doesn't share much about what he is feeling, I suggested that my husband just talk about general topics.

In terms of not knowing where all this is headed, our aunt said that she never wanted to go to a nursing home, ever. Nobody expected her to get Alzheimer's, so this is a different decision now. They are devoted to her and will need to make a good decision about the future keeping the reality of the situation in mind. We want them to know that they can count on us to listen to them and support them until they can't do it anymore.

Kellie talks about her devotion to her grandfather

Of course I felt committed to my grandfather's care and was completely devoted to him as a person. I felt that this was my only choice. Even when I put my Grandfather in the nursing home after his stroke, I was still very involved. Once I commit I am definitely there for the long haul regardless of the outcome.

Musings on Mayeroff:

Caring grows over time and is impacted by the stressors of life, and devotion is especially manifested by "being there" through the difficulties that Caregivers face.[11]

Author's reflections:
It is often said that Caregiving is not for the faint of heart. Out of the challenge comes a shared experience that holds the possibility of bringing people closer. Sitting together in a doctor's office waiting for test results is one such shared experience. Going through boxes and boxes of papers to find that one bank form from seven years ago is another shared experience. When the two of you mesh into a team of support and devotion even the bad news or lost forms are easier to handle.

A Caregiver who sticks around, faces challenges and is committed to filling the needs of the person being cared for achieves the ultimate in caring. There are many who aren't strong enough to "stick it out" but for those that do comes a strong sense of devotion and purpose. Others witness this devotion and wonder how it continues in the face of so much stress.

Do you feel sometimes that, by letting others see the stress you are under, they will know how committed you are to your Caregiving?

Debbie talks about not needing others to witness her devotion to her Caregiving

My sisters and I don't seem to need others in the family or the community to witness our Caregiving. We witnessed each other's devotion by sharing and acknowledging what we were doing for our mom. We would also validate our feelings of respect and care for each other. In that way, seeing my caring through their eyes helped me to define what it was that I was doing and the devotion I felt.

My husband's brother and sister-in-law don't need others to see their caring either. They aren't looking for praise. In our family it comes from the heart. They are devoted to our aunt without needing any credit for doing it.

There are people I know in my massage profession who glory in what they have done for their clients. They need the attention and take all the credit for healing. It's more about them and their great work and less about their client's place in the healing.

Kellie talks about her Caregiving being witnessed

I hadn't thought about it before but I do think that others in the community did see the devotion I had in caring for my family and were affected by it. I hope I inspired them.

I don't want to be put up on a pedestal, but if others are more confident about Caregiving because they saw me do it with my three relatives, I would love that. I know they saw me take on Caregiving for three people without hesitating in my devotion to them. I was committed to their care over many years.

Now when people in my life have similar situations and they are frightened and don't know what's next, I can help them. Caregiving becomes almost simple. It's about expressing your love and then finding the right number to call Medicaid for example. By getting the important things done, they can stay centered for the person they are caring for. Once they understand that it is all about true caring they can relax. Even when the challenges get in the way, they'll know to get back to their feelings of connection as the basis for their caring. I am happy that I could be a role model for that.

Has your devotion ever been an issue? Do you ever feel that you are holding yourself back, neglectful or ambivalent about your role as a Caregiver?

Debbie talks about holding back with her mother

Sometimes I would be ambivalent in practical ways like talking to my mom because I didn't want to get on the phone with her again. This ambivalence was more from my frustration because I wondered if my mom was ever going to listen to my suggestions or insights. Her actions showed me that she wasn't really open to changing in areas that I considered important. The frustration was the hesitation but it never made me question my devotion to her overall care.

It wasn't as hard to visit because she was glad to see me and I could tell more about her emotions. There was no hesitation when I saw her in person. It helped that she was more receptive to my ideas when we spoke face to face. I learned early on not to lecture her because it didn't work. It worked much better for me to listen and find out what she really was trying to say.

I realize now that technically I could have just walked away from the whole situation with my mom and let my sister handle everything. At the time I didn't feel ambivalent at all. It never even entered my consciousness to think about doing that.

In another practical matter we were all holding ourselves back in terms of her physical well-being. This wasn't because we weren't devoted to her or her health but more because we believed that she was being responsible. Just before she died we had started to wonder about what was really going on. She was still able to drive and make decisions, so on the surface things looked fine.

You can't force someone to get in their own car and drive themselves to the doctor's. The other problem with the way healthcare is set up is that the doctors won't call the family to tell them that she was canceling her appointments due to their privacy constraints. We wouldn't find these things out unless she told my aunt. Becoming more active in a situation like that was really hard but we were just starting to figure out how to deal with it.

I didn't feel ambivalent about taking care of my mother's finances. It was how I could show her that I was committed to reducing her stress by helping her become financially solvent. I found it easy to reassure her that I had paid the bill and hadn't paid too much or too little. This was her reality at the time to worry and ask.

None of these practical matters ever got in the way of my sisters and my dedication to our mother. We had a lot to learn about what we had taken on but our hearts were in the right place.

Kellie talks about the idea of holding back with her father and stepmother

I didn't hold back with my dad. I tend to give 110% in anything I do. I probably held back the most with my step-mother because she was more independent. I wasn't hesitating in my overall commitment but just in some practical matters. I was more hesitant with her because I didn't want to step on her toes and have her feel that she was losing her independence because of her cancer. I only held back because I was being considerate of her as the person she was. It was the right thing to do for as long as she could still do things herself.

Kellie talks about holding back with her grandfather

I did hold back in caring for my grandfather when he had his stroke. My instincts would have been to immediately go get him and bring him to our house. A lot of my friends also assumed that I would have him come and live with us. When I really thought about it though, I said no to this arrangement for his sake. I couldn't do that to him. He would have suffered too much.

At first I questioned my hesitation but then I really thought about it. He was happy in his home. He had all his friends there and everything he knows is there. In the end I felt that making arrangements for him to stay in his home was absolutely the right thing to do.

Author's reflections:
Being a Caregiver requires a great deal of flexibility to continue being devoted over the long haul. A Caregiver needs to be able to change plans and approaches to their care on the spur of the moment. Often we are asked to move beyond the engrained habits or basic personality traits we've gotten by on for our entire lives. We may almost feel that we've surrendered control of our whole way of being.

Would you describe your personality as flexible or driven? Give an example. Has your personality interfered with your sense of devotion?

Debbie talks about her flexibility while caring for her mother

I've always been flexible in terms of what I would share with my mother. I was able to delay my feeling of being annoyed until after I got off the phone. That way we could talk without fighting.

I've learned to carry this flexibility through to situations like dealing with my mom and her excessive cat adoptions. I tried to be flexible in how I approached the topic with her. Being logical and pointing out the downside of having all these cats were the ways I kept my horror and frustration hidden from her. I never let my judgments about her cat adoptions get in the way of my overall devotion to her.

There were times when the conversation didn't go as well as I wanted. I would be left with a feeling of frustration. That's when I would go to my husband who would be a good sounding board when I got upset. It never occurred to me to abandon my care for my mother in the midst of our differences. I tried to be flexible so I could continue with my Caregiving for her.

Debbie talks about being flexible as a parent

There is a natural devotion that comes with being a parent. I think just the choice to have a child starts the dedication to their life and the hopes of it working well for them. That being said, in order to keep my sanity as a parent I had to change my personality from being very judgmental of others to being more flexible.

With my son, especially when he was a teen, I had to be very flexible. It was important to pick my battles. I needed to understand what was important not just to me but to him as well. Adolescent angst can alter perceptions and give more weight to things that I may have thought meaningless. In order for me to remain devoted to his flourishing I needed to learn about him and the various stages he was going through.

I was more inflexible when I was younger. I did have to learn over the years that my high standards caused problems. I would hold others up to these standards and if they fell short I would judge them. I learned how to be more flexible by being a parent. It's not that I've lowered my standards but I have changed my expectations of others having to measure up to them.

I'm generally laid back now but I do still have strong values that I expect everyone to be following. In spite of that I've mellowed with age and my Yoga practice. It's not worth the energy to judge others and it gets in the way of true devotion.

Kellie talks about her own flexibility with her family

Most people think of me as flexible but I'm really not. I'm pretty stubborn and driven. Once I have something in my head that I'm working on I have a very difficult time changing course mid-stream. Being this way has never gotten in the way of my overall devotion to my caring and my relationships. They come first but sometimes it's hard.

An example was the day that I had to take my grandfather to the doctor. My ex-husband is completely flexible about changing plans and called to say we have to pick up our car today. As a result he informed me that we have to reschedule Grandpa's doctor's appointment. I flip out. In my head I've already taken him to the doctor, made dinner for him and it is all set.

My dad and step-mother were the same. If there was a plan, we wouldn't change it unless it was more than 24 hours in advance. It probably had something to do with my dad's role as a public speaker and an economist. He needed to be very organized and so do I. My real mom is like that too, very organized.

Musings on Mayeroff:
We don't know what the future holds, but we commit ourselves to the other person regardless.[12]

Author's reflections:
One of the hardest things that any of us have to handle is not knowing the future. We often live our lives assuming our expectations will bear out. For example: If I do A then B will follow; if I work I'll get paid, if I study I'll graduate, if I train at the gym I'll get stronger. In Caregiving the future is uncertain and we are required to jump in and help out anyway. When we commit to Caregiving, we are signing on to the care of another person and to the uncertainties that will follow as well.

How do you feel about not knowing where your Caregiving will take you? How does this affect your ability to remain devoted?

Debbie talks about not knowing the effect of moving her mother into town

Because of my spiritual practice and meditation I no longer have an expectation of how things will turn out. The overall commitment to my Caregiving stays strong. As soon as my mother moved into the rental house in town she was so much more relaxed that I never second-guessed myself or our decision. Things just got better and better for her during the last six months of her life.

Kellie talks about handling the uncertainties of the future

Not knowing the future is horrifying to me! I'm really bad with being flexible and I'm really bad with change. My grandpa who was very soft spoken would always try to convince me that change was the only constant in life. He thought this should be a comfort to me.

I was 19 years old and couldn't grasp this at all. I intellectually understood the concept but couldn't embrace the emotional experience of it. In reality my grandpa hated change too but he was trying to convince himself that he should embrace change as something good. He was very introspective and would be able to talk himself into things.

Not knowing how things will turn out is maddening to me. Even my new job is freaking me out. I'm scared of change even when there are very few unknowns. I already know my new boss and I'm doing the exact same work as before. I can walk to work now, I know the area very well and I still have fear about it. It seems to be in my nature to want certainty.

I have no problem remaining committed to my relationships and my Caregiving even though I have this personality that prefers certainty. My devotion never waivers but from day to day sometimes my life is bumpy when I don't know how things will turn out. That's just me!

Section B

What elements go into caring?

Chapter 4

Knowing another

Author's reflections:
There's a reason why hearsay isn't admissible as evidence in a court of law. When we base our opinion and what we know about a person on what others have told us, we are filtering that knowledge and opinion through another's eyes. We can have the best of intentions, but unless we experience someone for ourselves we aren't really able to say we know them.

I remember a couples' therapist saying that sometimes she feels as if there were four people in the relationship she is counseling: the two people she actually sees in her office, and the highly filtered images that they have created for her in their description of each other.

Musings on Mayeroff:
When we care for another we need to come to deeply know that person. When we know someone we don't only passively experience their existence but we actively inquire to learn more about them in their own right.[13]

Author's reflections:
Caregiving for a family member, friend, or neighbor begins with the relationship you had before you were called upon to become their Caregiver. How well you knew this person and their quirks, their strengths and weaknesses, how they view the world, and the unique way in which the two of you related to each other in the past, will all affect the nature of the caring relationship.

The simple feeling of loving someone is a good start, but not enough when called upon to be someone's Caregiver. Caregiving entails a significantly more complex relationship than simply loving or caring for someone. When you become a Caregiver it is important to understand how much of who you are as well as how your history with that person will color the reality of who that person truly is. It's also important to remain as objective as you can in learning more about them as you journey down the path of Caregiving together.

You will be changing in the process and so will they. Their reactions to what is happening to them, due to their frailty and the nature of being under care, will be very different from yours, and you may not always agree on a number of issues, especially with how that person is managing what little independence is left to them. There is a real need to sharpen our skills of observation and inquiry in order to learn more about the person we are caring for.

How well do you know the person you are caring for?

Christie talks about knowing her husband

My husband and I lived together for about 20 years before his Alzheimer's started to become obvious. I would say that I knew him very well. I would also add that we were very different in some important ways. I was much more outgoing and social and earlier on he was more of a loner and involved with his writing and music.

Before his Alzheimer's began we had worked out our differences. Because I knew him so well, and wasn't interested in changing him, I arranged to have my friends share my social life while he stayed home and worked. I would go out to eat or see a movie with these buddies of mine. I like to travel, and, to not deprive myself of the enjoyment, arranged to do much of it solo. He was happy to hear about my adventures and when I was home we were very close. We shared important interests like fitness and music and did many things together as well.

When he started to become more dependent on me as his Alzheimer's progressed, I was able to include all the things I knew about him in our interactions. Having him maintain his dignity was an important goal of mine and knowing him so well helped me anticipate his needs. I would use music, fitness and humor to help him stay connected to me and our world.

As I observed the progression of his Alzheimer's I also noticed many new things about him. Since he could no longer work, he started to look forward to going out. He began to be more social and loved going to the movies. As he changed I needed to adapt and plan differently. We now often visited together with my friends. He also began to like to travel and we took many trips together during his last eight years.

Joe P. talks about knowing his wife

I knew my wife well. I generally knew what was going on with her, but there were times I couldn't reach her. She was inflexible about certain beliefs. When she would get fixed and rigid about something it didn't surprise me.

In the end she knew that she was dying. Because I knew her deeply and now carefully observed her reactions to her cancer I knew she was very, very strong, that she had accepted that she was dying. I also knew she wanted to leave this life. I had learned about her strength earlier in our marriage and saw it play out during her last days.

Could you take care of someone you didn't know very well?

Christie talks about caring for the other residents in the nursing home

Caring for someone I didn't know very well would depend on the situation.

Christie and her husband.

I'm usually pretty good at listening and taking my cues from a person, even though I may not know them very well. It probably would more depend on whether the person lets me in.

When I would visit my husband in the nursing home I usually would get some kind of response from the people at his lunch table. He was living on the floor where everyone was either in the middle or later stages of Alzheimer's.

It depended on what time of the day I was able to visit. With "sun downing," a late afternoon restlessness that occurs in many with Alzheimer's, nothing I did would penetrate the collective anxiety and aggression of the residents. Even knowing my husband so well didn't help when he was experiencing "sun downing." That was frustrating for me and I tried to avoid visiting him in the late afternoon.

Joe P. talks about caring for someone he doesn't know

I learned that because of the experience of taking care of my wife, I am now able to take care of someone else even if I didn't know them as well. I've been able to do this in other areas besides failing health like with the people I have mentored. The experience of being a Caregiver for my wife really opened my heart to others and their difficulties.

Joe P. talks about caring for his younger friend

I experience a totally non-judgmental caring with my younger friend. He had spent summers with my wife and I during his teen years and just recently we reunited after a ten year break. I imagine that the feelings I have for him must be similar to the experience of when you have a child of your own. Because I feel this way about him, and even though I don't know him as well as I did my wife, I could do the same level of Caregiving with him without hesitation. Others call it unconditional love. It's the first time I ever experienced that and can express it to him now that he is an adult.

What about the Professional Caregivers like nurses and healthcare attendants? Do you think it is better for them when they know a great deal about their patients? How so?

Christie talks about others who cared for her husband knowing very little about him

I have mixed feelings about this. I was told by a nurse who used to work in a nursing home that it is better to let the staff experience your loved one as they are in the present. What I think she might have meant was that a family shouldn't keep focusing on who the person was before their illness (implying that that was the better version) and more on who they are becoming.

The staff seemed to connect to my husband right away in spite of the fact that they didn't really know much about him. I would follow the nurse's advice for the most part and join in my husband's recreation activities at the level that he was experiencing them with his Alzheimer's. At the same time, though, I would still do little things to remind the Professional Caregivers of who my husband had been hoping that this would help them respect him and his accomplishments and maybe form a deeper connection to him.

Joe P. talks generally about knowing patients better

I believe that it makes it easier on the Professional Caregiver to know the idiosyncrasies of their patients. That way they have more tools to deal with odd behaviors or stubbornness.

Is it important for the Professional Caregivers to know what the patient was like before their illness?

Christie talks about the nursing home staff knowing about her husband from before the illness

It must be difficult with Alzheimer's to imagine what the resident's life had been before the disease. I feel that sometimes it helps to give the professional a link to your loved one's past so they can understand their present behaviors or have more to share with them. I would often bring tapes of my husband's music and play them for the staff and the residents when he was in the nursing home. His previous musical ability impressed the staff and I think helped them to respect him more. They seemed to enjoy knowing more about him.

Joe P. talks about the hospital staff getting to know his friend/mentor

Yes, there is often a greater amount of respect for the patient when the staff knows more about them as a person and what they accomplished in their life.

When my mentor was dying in the hospital in Houston, an article had just come out about him in Runner's World. As it circulated through the staff and they realized who was lying in the room, the atmosphere changed completely. I saw the level of respect and reverence grow in the staff.

They now had an interest in him as a person that went beyond the patient/nurse relationship they had before. They talked to me about him and treated the family differently. Suddenly they were full of information about his condition, they answered questions, and they reassured us and his family that he was being cared for.

Musings on Mayeroff:
This depth of knowledge includes knowing their strengths and weaknesses, their needs and what will best enable them to flourish to the extent that they still are able.[14]

Author's reflections:
When a Caregiving journey begins, our immediate impulse is to try to learn a lot about the condition and the various treatment modalities the person we are caring for is facing. But what actually becomes more important over time is what we learn about them, ourselves, and our relationship with them. When we focus on our strengths and talents, their strengths and talents, and what makes the relationship flow, the Caregiving becomes more rewarding.

How does knowing the strengths and weaknesses of the person you are caring for enable you to do a better job? Describe how this might play out.

Christie talks about knowing the strengths and weaknesses of her husband

With Alzheimer's a person's strengths and weaknesses change over time. Once the progression of the disease began my husband became much more social. He also needed tasks to help him feel involved in life so I was always looking for things to occupy him. He became patient and could do things that required detailed work for long periods of time as long as they weren't complicated tasks. He helped out in the garden and with other tasks like food preparation, gathering kindling for the wood burning stove and laundry.

In the later stages his anxiety grew and he wasn't as motivated to stay busy so I had to adjust. I could no longer ask him to help with many of the tasks he had been happy to do before. That was much harder for me. In a way the progression of his disease became his weakness.

It was up to me to remember that the symptoms of Alzheimer's such as lethargy, were often what I was seeing and not his core qualities. I imagined that being overwhelmed with confusion must have been exhausting for him and the lethargy might have at least partly come out of that fatigue.

Joe P. talks about knowing his wife's strengths and weaknesses

My wife's strength was her intelligence. I knew that with her brilliance as long as she had her wits about her I should allow her to make the decisions she needed to make about her healthcare. Just because she was sick with cancer she could still make her own decisions about her treatment. I also appreciated that no matter whether she was in pain or not feeling well she could still focus, know what she wanted, and deal with what was needed at the time.

Her weaknesses revolved around the unresolved emotional issues with her family. She needed to prove something to them. She also allowed herself to be weak and dependent with them. Because I knew her and what the circumstances were I kept myself in check. It often meant my having to work around her issues with her family. Sometimes it was important not to say anything. I decided to deal with any of the negative fallout from her dependency on her family later.

Musings on Mayeroff:

Words aren't enough when it comes to describing what we experience of another. We can know each other beyond what words can convey. Knowing another can be both on an intuitive as well as cognitive level.[15]

Author's reflections:

There are literally thousands of love songs: we keep trying to find the best words to describe our loving feelings towards each other. Sometimes it's the music itself that does more to evoke the romantic feelings we mean to convey.

The same can be said of how we generally describe someone. Words can be hard to find or feel inadequate. "He's really sweet" or "she's a good person" don't demonstrate much depth.

Many Caregivers live in a world where spoken language almost doesn't matter. Just a look or movement from the person they are caring for can communicate volumes to a Caregiver. Sometimes just entering a room is enough to catch a vibe from someone in pain or who is feeling anxious about something. Words then take a back seat, and intuition and body language take over.

Give an example of how you know your loved one intuitively, without words. How are they different from you?

Christie talks about intuitively knowing her husband, though they were very different people

Once his Alzheimer's disease had progressed to the point where my husband was losing his verbal skills, I felt that I knew him in the same way that I know my birds. I would collect clues and make educated guesses about what he needed. Even though there were many things that I was able to guess at and infer, I would always have to check his response to see if I had gotten it right or at least close enough.

Earlier on he would put together a few words as he tried to communicate something to either myself or a friend. From these few words I was able to usually catch the drift of what he wanted to say. I became his translator.

The issue with intuition became more central as he lost most of his verbal abilities. At that point I was able to get my clues from guessing, thinking of our previous history or body language. Since there was less feedback, though, I wasn't sure that I was as in tune with him anymore.

The last year that he was in the nursing home, when the weather was nice, I would take him outdoors to walk the grounds or the garden path. I based this on an intuitive idea that he would enjoy being outside, seeing nature, having a change of scenery. Since we had done so, so many things outdoors in the earlier days of our relationship, I could only guess that he would enjoy this way of spending our time together.

In terms of our differences, my husband's intelligence drifted away with his Alzheimer's. He found pleasure in the simple things. Often I would bike ride with my friend. My husband was still able to ride along with us. She and I would be discussing the complex ideas related to acupuncture or some other topic, and he would pull us back to the simplicity of the moment. He would point to the turtles sunning themselves on a rock or the swans tending to their babies. Both of us appreciated his gentle reminders to stay focused on the ride and the enjoyment of the moment.

Joe P. talks about intuitively knowing his wife and their differences

During our marriage I knew immediately when my wife was in a situation she didn't like because she would shut down and say, "Let's get out of here." She had difficulty dealing with anyone who was less intelligent than her. I knew this about her without anything being said.

I'm different from her because if I need to suffer a fool I can do it and thereby make the best of the situation. Even though we were very different I still could understand how she was intuitively.

Musings on Mayeroff:
We must know ourselves as well as the person we are caring for, and know what strengths and weakness we each bring to this experience.[16]

Author's reflections:
Caregiving can be as much of a challenge to our self-image as what we do for a living or how we are as a parent. In these aspects or our lives we find out if we can handle a number of situations, both actual and emotional. When we discover our strengths and use them to their fullest, life seems to glide along.

On the other hand, it is often harder work to identify our natural weaknesses and then work on overcoming them. This honesty in knowing our weaknesses is an extraordinary burden which many Caregivers seem to think they can tackle on their own. In the end they may find their failed efforts have contributed to an already stressful situation. We all need to learn that it is okay to seek and get support, professional and otherwise, in trying to understand and overcome our shortcomings and how they relate to our Caregiving experience.

How have you brought your strengths and weaknesses into your caring? What are you good at? What has been hard for you?

Christie talks about her strengths and weaknesses in caring for her husband

During the eight years I was my husband's Caregiver my various strengths came out at different times. Since I'm a jazz musician I incorporated my ability to improvise from moment to moment in my approach to helping him stay within his skill levels.

I would often catch myself in the middle of a routine that we had performed a million times and realize quickly that it wouldn't work anymore to continue the way we had. This happened over time with his ability to get dressed, cook, do laundry, help around the house and garden. I needed to change the routine and change it quickly. I also needed to think outside the box to find solutions to problems as they arose. My jazz background helped with all of that flexibility.

I was constantly being called on to alter his tasks or help out when needed and usually I didn't miss a beat. What was hard were the times I could see that I would have to take over a task completely. This meant adding another chore to my already long list of jobs. To this day I still resent the jobs that I had labeled "hubbie's work."

Another strength I have is the remarkable amount of patience I have. Of course I would eventually break down and become irritable but that was only when I was already tired or stressed. It was hard to worry about financial matters and keep two homes and one office going while being generous and patient. I would say in the majority of cases I succeeded but not always.

Another strength I have is my ability to catch myself when I am becoming rigid and judgmental. For some reason I am able to be flexible and open to most of the symptoms of Alzheimer's, and I allowed the disease to challenge my pre-conceived ideas about truth, sanity, perspective, memory and reality. I loved comparing what we accept as "normal" to the new perspectives that came with this alteration of my husband's brain.

What became hard was his anxiety in the later stages of the disease, the repetitive questions and the restlessness especially his wandering around at night when I needed to sleep. This is what finally caused me to consider putting him in a nursing home for his last year and a half.

Another strength I have is being a very optimistic person in general. As we noticed my husband's symptoms in the early stages I was convinced that his was experiencing the non-progressive type of dementia. This idea comforted me for the first five years of his illness. As his symptoms got worse in stages I finally had to admit that he probably had the classic symptoms of Alzheimer's.

What made it hard was my inability to ask for help as I started to need it. I finally had no choice and my stubbornness melted into a whole community of professional help where I learned about the programs and resources that were available to us.

Joe P. talks about his strengths and weaknesses as he cared for his father

When I am Caregiving I don't find anything hard. My strength is that I always find ways of doing what I have to do. Because it comes from a very deep place and comes from my heart, I find it easy to care for someone. It has nothing to do with logic, if this person needs help I will help. No matter how crazy it gets in terms of circumstances I won't let it affect my caring.

My father's obstinacy was hard for me to handle and would annoy me at first. I judged it in a negative way. My judgment came out of my not yet fully understanding who he was. Once I saw his stubbornness as his strength it helped me to tolerate it and work with it, even when it came to be a threat to his well-being.

In my thirties I was much more judgmental but I'm not that way now. I've grown tremendously in the last 5 – 10 years and been able to live and let live. This growth coincided with caring for my father.

Chapter 5

Learning what comes of our caring and tweaking, always tweaking

Musings on Mayeroff:
Caregiving involves a feedback loop. By this we mean that it lets us see the effects of our actions as we care for another. The care we give can cause a range of reactions in the other person from joy to upset. Based on what we find we refine our behavior to better assist the other person's ability to flourish.[17]

Author's reflections:
This is the missing link for most of us. Thinking that what we do will help another person inspires us to act. Once we have taken this action we need to then stop and question whether our intervention really had the effect we intended it to have.

An example would be that you might want mom to get out more. She has some dementia and the doctor said she needs more stimulation. If she gets upset in your car, asks where you are taking her and seems anxious, combative and tries to open the door, maybe you haven't yet found the way to follow your doctor's orders. Next you try to take her for a walk up and down the street where her house is and everything is familiar. During your walk she gets a chance to talk to neighbors and you can tell by her demeanor that she is relaxed and enjoying the experience. Voila! You were able to learn what she likes and tweak the plan to suite her. She's happy and so are you and so is her doctor. As this example shows one way to evaluate the outcomes of your Caregiving, is to take note of whether the person seems positively energized by your actions.

Caregiving is about learning to find what works and tweaking it until you are successful. We may inadvertently be stepping into areas the other person would rather we weren't involved in, or we may not be doing enough for a person who needs a good deal more of our help. In either case, they may shrink back into seeming lethargy. A positive energy level in the person we are caring for is usually a good sign of positive Caregiving. Positive interventions often inspire the other person to move ahead with their lives or take on a brighter outlook, despite their difficulties.

Have you been able to change your approach when something isn't working? Give an example. How did the person in your care experience this?

Chris F. talks about being able to change while he cared for his mother who, at the same time, was caring for his father

My mother was in a very strong state of denial about my father's condition of Alzheimer's. This was back in the mid-90's when they didn't know as much about the disease as they do now. Ronald Reagan was around and admitted having Alzheimer's but many doctors didn't even acknowledge the disease. There still is no real diagnosis until after someone dies.

My dad had dementia but he would also have days of clarity so my mother thought he wasn't trying hard enough to be his old self. He was already in his 80's so she thought it might be a matter of his just being a bit forgetful. The word 'dementia' wasn't a part of peoples' vocabulary back then. 'Senility' was used but it was used loosely.

My father's case went far beyond a little forgetfulness. The first doctor we went to didn't think there was anything to worry about. It was only when my father went to the hospital and saw a doctor with more experience that they finally diagnosed his Alzheimer's disease.

Even after his diagnosis my mom never really understood that there was no cure for Alzheimer's. In her mind she felt it was a phase he was going through and he would snap out of it. We are talking about a large man, over 6 feet and 225 pounds who was becoming at best an adolescent. She would get upset with him and act like what he was doing was his fault. We would argue about how she was talking to him. She would talk at him and expect him to do whatever she said the same way you might talk to a bad child or a pet. She did it out of love but she didn't have the capacity to understand what was happening to my father. You have to remember that this man had been her rock. Now the pendulum had swung and she was required to be more like a mother again.

I was basically arguing that I had to clean up the emotional mess she was making. The fact that I was her son made it hard for her to appreciate what I was saying. She was accusing me of being coldblooded and hammering her and I'm accusing her of ignorance and lack of competence. I got so involved because I was living with them at the time. None of this was working but I hadn't understood that I needed to learn how to better care for not only my father but also for my mother regardless of her lack of Caregiving skills.

What made me seriously have to alter my approach to her was when one day my father saw us arguing. On this particular day he said "Please stop fighting, I'll be good." That hit me really hard. I went to the basement and cried like a baby. What I learned was that he had thought that our arguing and upset was all his fault. Of course I later told him it wasn't his fault.

In that single moment I learned the irony of what was happening. Here I was arguing with her about berating him, and now I saw how I was treating her and that was even worse. I felt guilty about it because I felt that I should have known better.

From what I learned that day I changed my approach to my mom. I was very aware of what I would say before I said anything. I became aware of her reaction to my words. I had been like that before all of this started but because of my dad's Alzheimer's I now needed an extra degree of sensitivity to her. I realized that none of this was easy for her and she was suffering. I started to see how this whole situation was affecting everyone so even when I felt she was wrong I had to accept it.

I also learned that some of my arguing came from my own frustration and anger. I had been upset that my mother hadn't gone to the right doctor in the beginning and also she had delayed my father's being able to retire. She didn't know what he would do with himself with all that free time and worried that he might lose his motivation. He was a full time minister in his 80's. I blamed her at the time but I didn't realize that she was being supportive in her own way. It was hard for me to see but gradually I learned to see her side of things and changed how I treated her.

In the end I had to subdue my anger to navigate their peace. It was a big change for me because I'm used to speaking my mind. I had to finally realize that this was an area that no one could be perfect in. Once we stopped raising our voices my father became generally less agitated and he could listen better to what my mother was asking of him. She was also much calmer because I was no longer jumping down her throat. Between me and her we still had a cold war that simmered under the surface but better that than the fighting.

I also connected the fact that during this whole time I at least had a job so I could have a break. My mother took all this on willingly and was there all the time for my dad. I started to appreciate that my mother cared deeply for my father and I'm sure this whole thing took years off of her life.

When I spoke at his funeral I told everyone that she had done the best she could and that she had nothing to feel guilty about. I don't know for sure, but I hope that she heard what I said and that it hopefully made her feel a little better about herself.

Susan talks about her needing to change while caring for her husband

I think I am doing well with my Caregiving because I've learned I can change things in many practical ways as we go along. For instance, my husband, who has early-onset Alzheimer's, was having trouble pulling his chair up to the table so I got him an office chair on wheels. Now he can easily move his chair himself. When he was having trouble with snapping and zipping his jeans, I got him elastic waist sweat pants that he can pull on himself. I have found that when I've learned how to find a solution to one of his issues, my husband seems to be relieved and can experience less frustration.

Also on a practical level, since we have a large two-story house, I learned that we would have to change things around somewhat to keep things running smoothly. After trying a few things, I have set up the upstairs for myself

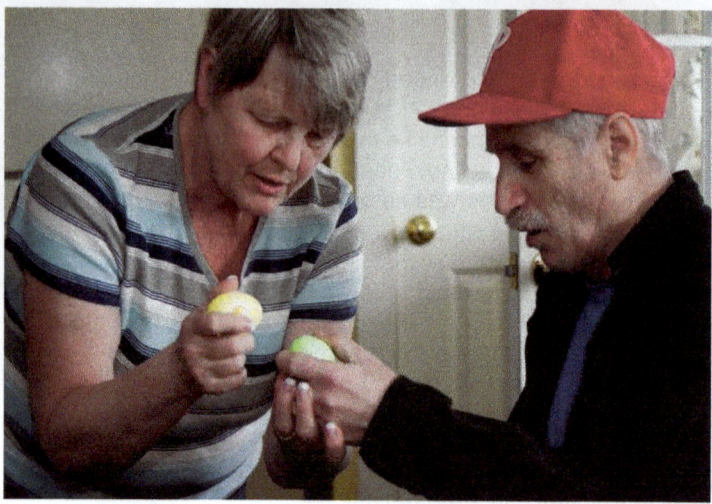

Susan and her husband.

and our young grandsons and created a bedroom downstairs for my husband. It allows us to keep his space a bit calmer and quieter so he can relax without getting frustrated and startled.

I was concerned that I might not know when he needs assistance, especially during the night, so I set up a video monitor in his bedroom that I can observe from my room upstairs. This allows me to check on him at any moment and know when he needs assistance. It allows me to sleep more comfortably knowing I can hear or see him anytime. It also avoids anxiety for him because I can get to him quickly before he panics about anything. It's been a lot of learning and tweaking but I'm happy with the way things are going for all of us. There's a lot of positive energy in our family right now.

Author's reflections:
Being flexible in our thinking and agile in our actions helps us to avoid being dogmatic. It is easy to slip into patterns and habits of thought that become rigid and unbending. In our caring we need to admit when things just aren't going well and be willing to try new options.

Musings on Mayeroff:

Sometimes doing nothing seems to be the best course when dealing with another person in a caring capacity. Not giving an opinion, not agreeing or disagreeing, sometimes is the best way to help another. Of course, monitoring the effect of doing nothing will help us to see if this truly has been the best course to take and perhaps inform the plan should a similar situation arise in the future.[18]

Author's reflections:
This is a skill that we are never taught in school: the skill of inaction. Most of our world is made up of a flurry of activities and we get swept along.

But sometimes a situation calls for inaction instead of action. Taking a deep breath, waiting, listening and observing are all choices available to us in Caregiving situations. Stepping back and taking cues from the other person is sometimes the best thing we can do for them. The challenge will be theirs and so will discovery and growth. At the same time, we need to be monitoring the effects of our inaction with the aim of determining whether it has led to positive outcomes.

Have you ever opted to do or say nothing in a caring situation? What were the effects? What was the response from the other person? Have you tried it again?

Chris F. talks about stepping back with his ex-fiancée

To tell you the truth, I may have stated my piece and then stepped away to see how someone would react, but I can't ever remember doing nothing at all. It's not my style.

An example of this was when I stepped away after stating my piece with my ex-fiancée. She and I had already broken up. The next guy she ended up going out with was a bum in my opinion. Shortly after I had found out about him we went out to dinner. Because I still cared for her I told her that I felt that this relationship wasn't good for her. Once I spoke my piece I barely spoke to her on the way home and that was that.

In terms of our relationship we didn't speak for a long time after that. I heard about her from her family but never directly from her. I felt that that was the price I was willing to pay for my honesty. I needed to let her learn the lessons of life and by not doing anything after my comments to her. I felt that I was allowing her to struggle and grow.

I would do and have done the same thing in other situations. I feel that after I give my opinion it is really up to the other person to act. If I take action then they don't get a chance to learn and grow because they are merely reacting to me and my actions.

Susan talks about when she chooses to say nothing with her husband

Because of his dementia, I frequently say nothing to my husband when I feel it would be too overwhelming for him. Instead of telling him of our plans as they are being formulated I wait. I have several strategies. I might wait to tell him of an upcoming event such as a doctor's appointment or someone coming to visit until the night before and then again the morning of.

If I tell him too long ahead he forgets. I might just tell him the short version of what is happening. If I give him too much information at one time, he gets confused and overwhelmed. Sometimes if I begin a conversation and he seems confused about it, I stop and try again later when he seems less confused or frustrated.

Chapter 6

Rhythm of switching back and forth from the big picture and the individual moment

Musings on Mayeroff:
Sometimes Caregiving requires seeing an individual situation in a more panoramic way. A step back in order to see the whole picture allows us to take into consideration past, future, and peripheral aspects of that person's care; helping us to then make better decisions for them.[19]

Author's reflections:
Often we need to take a giant step back in order to see the whole picture of a relationship. Children who are taking care of frail or sickly parents carry the entire history of their relationship into their Caregiving.

When dealing with the intensity of what Caregiving can become certain behaviors can become infuriating. A parent who is stubborn, selfish or anxious on a daily basis can be very hard on the person giving the care. Small things can turn into arguments or ongoing frustrations. Not wanting to go to the senior center or not wanting to go out at all can be hard on the Caregiver. How do you get someone to the doctor when they refuse to leave the house?

To find the patience it often helps to switch to thinking about the big picture of the situation. Some of these daughters or sons think about what their parents have given them over the span of their life and feel that now it is their time to give back. They remember the nice times they had in order soften their hearts as they feel themselves getting annoyed. Others think about the rough childhood that their parents endured and to compensate for their suffering want them to find some joy in their remaining years. They may use humor to coax mom or dad out the door to help "those old folks" at the senior center. And then there are those who have had a difficult relationship with their parents and see the big picture of their own future. They care for their parent simply to alleviate any guilt they might feel if instead they were to choose to neglect their relative. This is the most difficult way of looking at things because the motivation is to take care of themselves more than their parent. However sometimes this is the best that can be done in a situation.

Give an example of a Caregiving situation you were in where looking at the "big picture" saved the day.

Keith talks about looking at the "big picture" with his son

The big picture is that I often go to the AA meetings with my oldest son. Someday I'm hoping that he'll understand the big picture of this disease that he's involved with. I wish that he'll use the others at the meetings as role models and inspiration when he's ready to change. I believe that someday the stories he hears there will finally sink in. At the meetings people share how they were down and clawed themselves back up. I know when you are 21 you feel immortal but the big picture shows us that, as time goes on, people change and grow. He hasn't realized that yet. He has his whole life in front of him.

When I think about the long term in ten years he'll either keep doing what he's doing and possibly be dead or he will have come to grips with his life and gotten himself together. He may end up married to his girlfriend and since he is quite talented maybe someday he'll be able to apply his talents to some kind of work. He's a real people person and hopefully that will somehow save him.

Keith talks about the big picture of caring for his wife

The big picture in terms of caring for my wife as she deals with our sons from day to day is that I can help her feel that she is not alone. She has me to care for her and I do my best to give her everything she needs to support her. Since I work I can't be there to do the constant monitoring that is required to keep our sons out of trouble but I can be there for her as her support.

I really can't imagine Caregivers who are trying to do all of this alone, whether it be an elderly parent or someone who's sick or a couple of kids who are addicted to drugs. It's so much easier when you have someone to share the experience with.

Because my wife is in this abusive situation as the main Caregiver for our two sons, I feel that it is my role to take care of her as best I can. The normal thing that happens is the kids lie to her or don't call or don't take their medications and she gets upset. I feel that my job is to try to calm her down but especially to let her vent and listen without judgment.

The big picture in the midst of all the individual dramas is that this is what she needs from me. She has no one else she can talk to and sometimes she needs to go on and on about something. I may even have a better overview of what is really happening but it's important for me to let her have her say and not interrupt. I sometimes feel like I'm some kind of therapist. I can't imagine if something were to happen to me how she would handle everything.

Liz talks about seeing the big picture with her mother-in-law

The first thing I learned about the big picture was that you have to decide whether you want to get involved in Caregiving. As long as you do it from the heart and the person is asking you to do the caring, then it's OK. Otherwise it can be condescending or patronizing to think we know better and barge in uninvited.

The next thing I learned about the big picture for me was that I learned to accept the situations I couldn't change. We cared for my mother-in-law as a family. I was a big part of her Caregiving team and later was a frequent visitor. She started showing signs of dementia after several strokes and was addicted to several medications. Her husband had been a pharmacist and had provided her with various medications over the years. When she was dropped into our lives and lived with us for three months the doctor advised us to get her off of everything.

My friend who is a nurse described a situation where an 85 year-old alcoholic was told that she couldn't live with her children if she continued to drink and she stopped in one day. I thought there might be hope for my mother-in-law. The difference is that she didn't want to stop her narcotics and pain-killers and that makes all the difference. She kept screaming at us to give her the black bag with all her medications.

I don't know what her oldest daughter was thinking at the time but it seemed like she just wanted to let her mother keep taking her medications. Maybe she was considering the big picture that her mother had been doing these drugs for so many years and didn't want to stop now. She went with her mother to one doctor after another until they found someone who agreed that she should keep taking everything. Just as an aside, what was truly horrible was that in the end my mother-in-law was in a lot of pain, but because the pain medicine was no longer working for her there was nothing anyone could do. That was a difficult experience for us to go through with her.

My husband's older sister was the head of the Caregiving team and the go to person for decisions. My husband was involved and they would speak often. I would also be there and went to the family meetings with the social worker who was guiding us on what we would have to do and when.

I observed that my husband's brother's wife was inserting herself heavily in the talks, asking questions and giving her opinions. My husband came away with a negative opinion about what she was doing. He didn't feel it was appropriate for her to be so involved since she was only related to his mother by marriage. From these comments I knew my place as being in the same role. I also knew there was no payoff in going to battle with the older sister.

I would have liked my husband to be stronger when it came to his sister, but I realized there was a family dynamic and hierarchy at work. I never asked him to stand up to her but this meant there were times when things didn't go my way or my husband's way. He mostly just wanted to avoid conflict. For example, his sister chose an assisted living facility for their mother that was a much further drive for us. I was hoping that he would object because I was the one going over there the most. This was because everyone else was working. During that same time I wasn't working because I was caring for my kids while they were in school. He didn't speak up to her so I had to make the longer trip each way.

The big picture is that we wanted to come out intact at the end of this whole affair. We still wanted to be a family and relate to his family and that was the most important thing to us. It worked because we all still get along to this day. The fact that everybody took their places and I bit my tongue made it all work.

I understood this dynamic while we were going through the situation. Even in a marriage you have to pick your battles and I would never ask someone to go up against their siblings or their parents unless they initiated it.

I associate looking at the big picture with focusing on what your overall goals are as you acquire wisdom in certain situations. I learned when to hold back my feelings so my marriage and family relationships would continue on past any difficulties we might be having at a particular time or in a particular circumstance.

Musings on Mayeroff:
Sometimes separating one event out from the larger picture and reflecting on it as a stand-alone event is the best way to approach a situation.[20]

Author's reflections:
When we approach our Caregiving in a way that puts the emphasis on each chore, each sweet moment, one day at a time, we save ourselves from being overwhelmed by the larger picture. Putting one foot in front of the other seems doable in a world that is rapidly changing into something new and strange. The losses don't feel as harsh when we concern ourselves with the mundane tasks of life like laundry and meal preparation.

This approach can also work for behaviors. Sometimes it is easier to forgive or be patient with something that was only done once or seems to not fit the norm. When someone has cancer and the treatment is giving them "chemo brain" their forgetting to pick up the milk is more understandable. When a diabetic normally takes care of themselves but suddenly starts getting irritable because they don't have the proper food available one day, we can better understand and ignore their harsh words.

Was there ever a time when you saw a behavior as just a one- time, isolated occurrence? Did that throw you off the track from your usual way of caring for that person?

Keith talks about the behavior of his younger son who is addicted to drugs and alcohol

I wish I could think of something but by now my sons have repeated the same behaviors over and over again. Whether it is lying, or stealing our money or credit cards, we've seen it all before. We try to be pre-emptive but it's the one time we forget and don't lock the bedroom door or leave the purse on the counter or whatever, that they find their opportunities and take advantage.

In terms of a onetime positive event, we did hear from one of our youngest son's counselors that our child was amazing in this one group program he went to for 6 weeks. It was about coping with life skills. The counselor said he was helpful to him and the other kids and he was sociable, which is difficult for him with the Asperger's, a mild form of Autism. My wife and I were on top of the world. We thought for sure we were on our way to a "normal" life. We had never gotten such a good report from anyone in his life before. This was definitely different from his usual behaviors. Sadly he went back to his old behaviors after he finished the program.

There was also a period of time that was unusual for him. He was in his fifth year of high school and after lawsuits and court cases we were successful in getting him the support he needed at school. They finally put him in a smaller class. He started to thrive and the teacher was even asking him to help the other kids. This was extra special in that he had come into the course late. Again, my wife and I were thrilled at such a difference from his normal behavior and again he reverted back once school ended.

They had an astronomy course at night for star-gazing, and my son was leaving an hour early to get there so I asked him about it. He said he was helping the teacher set up. When I asked his teacher he said that my son was his number one student. These reports were all rare for him. They kept us going for quite a while each time. Even though these positive reports were merely a brief break from his usual troubling patterns, we finally had some hope. Now that he has been involved in drugs it gets harder to continue to hope but we do.

Liz talks about only being able to see the big picture in her and her mother's Caregiving experiences

I wish I could have seen certain behaviors as one time occurrences. It would have given me a chance to forgive and forget. Instead I can't think of anything where certain behaviors weren't linked to the big picture or repeated themselves over and over. We didn't have a break and I never had a chance to say "Oh, but that was only that one time, so it's OK and hopefully it won't happen again." That would have been great.

My mother-in-law who had Alzheimer's, was always asking for her drugs and this kept going until the very end of her life. My husband's whole family kept her big picture in mind as they consulted with each other and avoided confrontations with her. Nobody thought of her behaviors as a one-time occurrence. They had seen the same things over and over.

The same thing was true for my mother. She had the grueling task of caring for my dad who was frail and had dementia. They were in a routine that happened again and again so that was her big picture. There was seldom anything unique that happened. Even his "sundowning" which made him extremely irritable and suspicious towards the end of the day got to be expected and part of the big picture. But again my mom had no relief and couldn't say that one of my dad's behaviors was a onetime occurrence. It made hope hard when things would happen over and over. Having something change gives a sense of possibilities but she didn't have that.

Chapter 7

Patience in caring

Author's reflections:
We all know that impatience can add strain to a relationship. When illness or disability strike, patience is one of the most important lessons to be learned by both parties. For the Caregiver it's a matter of having patience for the new level of function as is the case after a stroke or an automobile accident. It could be about having patience with the behavioral issues that pop up with mental illness, addictive behaviors or dementia. Remembering that these are symptoms related to illness or disability helps.

The person with the issues needs patience with themselves as they navigate new ways of doing things, learning new skills, and acquiring the ability to cope with it all. They also need patience with a partner who may be struggling to understand what they are feeling and searching for a balance in their Caregiving, avoiding doing too much, being hyper-vigilant or at other times not doing enough.

Even after two people have lived in a harmony of bio-rhythms, when illness strikes, discordance may arise. Often the Caregiver, who may be speedy about things, will need to wait for the other to dress, walk, get into and out of cars, or finish eating. When we Caregivers become frustrated or impatient we may be setting the entire relationship off kilter. The person we are caring for may feel badly for their inability to move faster, and we may be feeling upset and guilty for prodding them into a pace they can't match.

We each have a tempo that we are comfortable with. Some of us travel slowly through life and others seem to always be riding in the fast lane.

In a Caregiving situation, it is almost always the Caregiver whose time and habits are imposed upon. But when we commit to caring, we are also committing to adjust our tempo to that of those we are caring for. When we do this we can feel gratified, in synch, and we get to "smell the roses," bolstering the other's dignity and desire to do the best under the circumstances.

Musings on Mayeroff:
When we give fully of ourselves and actively participate with another, we give them time and space to explore and live.[21]

Author's reflections:
In order to fully and successfully care for another person, we must be giving of ourselves. Our giving can take many forms: money, time, chores, and of course our patience. Patience, as an intangible, may, for some, be the most difficult thing to give, especially when tested by the seemingly irrational behaviors of those in our care. With dementia, for example, we may lose patience if the person we are caring for cannot understand our words. With

cancer they may be too tired or weak to respond to us. With mental illness they may not have the ability to do what we are asking of them.

Sometimes our impatience overtakes our better judgment even before we realize it; but if we can somehow remain patient, we reward both ourselves and the person under our care. The partnership between Caregiver and those they are caring for becomes stronger with no damage done to either's feelings. At the same time, seeing the positive outcome in the one we are caring for helps us to tame our impatience, which may reinforce our more tolerant behavior, and thus strengthen the relationship even further.

What is the effect of rushing the person you are caring for? How do they respond?

Christie talks about the reasons not to rush her husband

Generally I knew that rushing my husband wasn't going to work. I would only slip into the need to rush my husband when we had an appointment. I would try to leave plenty of time to get everything done but there were often surprises, like a last minute visit to the bathroom, or shoes being on the wrong feet. I could feel myself starting to get impatient and it would change the sound of my voice. Talking faster or louder or with more anger made everything worse. He would get upset, make more mistakes and I would see how everything was actually taking longer. Sometimes I'd catch myself and change my manner and other times I'd work myself into a snit that would last for a good part of the day.

I think that rushing someone, even myself, creates stress and is just as likely to interfere with progress as help. There is nothing about the disease that allows the person with Alzheimer's to get things done faster. They can have difficulty with verbal directions, they might have trouble locating things in space; even remembering what the task was in the first place can be a problem.

For me as a Caregiver, being patient in the face of all that was difficult. Depending on my energy levels, other things that were going on in my life and how much control I felt I had in the situation, my levels of patience would vary. My husband could sense these levels of either frustration or patience and he would respond in kind. When I would get upset so would he and when I managed to stay calm he would mostly follow suit.

Sarah talks about her Caregiver support group

The Caregivers in the support group that I facilitate seem to have an unusual amount of patience, which was surprising when coupled with the stress of caring for someone with cancer. Patience can also be about making decisions and planning. Waiting for someone to make an important decision about their health for example, especially when they don't want to do what is seen as best for them, can be difficult.

Their impatience appeared more regularly around the small details of their life. They would get upset at the person they were caring for because they hadn't taken the dirty dishes to the kitchen after having eaten a meal that was prepared for them. Since they didn't often show their impatience in an open way it was hard for me to know how the person they were caring for reacted to their impatience.

Sheri talks about what happens when she rushes her partner

If I rush her she gets angry, frustrated, off balance and then it backfires in my face. She can only be who she is and I'm trying to make her someone who she isn't. I used to try to rush her a lot because I move much quicker than her.

I know I can be patient because when I was with my grandmother or great grandmother I had more patience. I could accept their need to do things more slowly. I found that it was different in my relationship with my partner and I didn't have the same patience with her at first. I couldn't understand her need to do things slowly as well.

I've been able to change and grow with this. To help me not start feeling impatient I find things to do while she is getting ready. Or I change my expectation and when she says she's ready I know we are still another ten minutes away from leaving. I wait until she has her shoes on and is walking out the door to finally put my projects away and I still get to the car ahead of her. This way I haven't rushed her and I don't get upset because I'm not standing around waiting. I hate waiting with nothing to do. It's one of my pet peeves.

Author's reflections:
Claustrophobia is the fear of being closed into a small space or a fear that you won't be able to get out of a closed space. Emotionally we can experience this closed in feeling when someone is showing their impatience. We no longer have the time and space to explore, experience or continue our journey in our own way. Often this kind of pressure can cause us to fumble, be self-conscious and make mistakes.

When we have the gift of time and space we can feel inspired, creative and this in turn allows us greater perspective to solve problems, and be more productive.

Do you actually accomplish what you set out to do when you hurry the person you are caring for?

Christie talks about rushing her husband

Unless I was stressed and not paying attention I soon learned that rushing my husband would confuse and upset him because of his progressing Alzheimer's disease. If the goal was to get dressed and out of the house, rushing him made things worse. When I could I left extra time to do things and time for myself to stay relaxed. Having him upset, anxious and frustrated could be avoided if we took our time with things.

I can easily see that one problem for the Caregiver of someone with Alzheimer's, mental illness or addictive behaviors is that the person seems to be doing things on purpose. Slow reactions, lack of initiative and confusion could all be interpreted as laziness or worse.

Patience kept the reality of my husband's situation front and center for me. Remembering the vast constellation of symptoms that were involved with Alzheimer's helped me stay patient most of the time. I saw that he wasn't doing things like putting his pants on backwards to frustrate me on purpose. When I rushed him his skill levels would immediately go down and everything took longer to do. I'd end up cleaning up spills or leaving the house without important papers. It never helped to rush him.

Sheri talks about rushing her partner

No, rushing her never works. I've learned how to adjust myself to her rhythms. If I rush her we both end up getting upset and it feels like it is taking her even longer to get ready.

Author's reflections:
When there is impatience, either theirs or ours, we are actually losing quality time. Although this may seem counter-intuitive, and it would seem that if we went faster, we'd get more done in less time. What actually happens is that we are working harder but not smarter and usually less is getting done.

What do you experience when you are being rushed?

Christie talks about herself outside of her Caregiving

I get crazed when I am being rushed, even by my own self-imposed deadlines. I make mistakes, forget things and often I take longer to do things. I do my best to have lots of time in situations, like planning ahead and arriving early. I often feel that I'm in some sort of zone when my internal rhythms match my activities.

When I am being pushed too fast I no longer match my own flow and this makes me crazy. On a small scale this same thing happens when I am playing music at our rehearsals. There is a speed for each tune that feels comfortable and beyond that it is no longer music but a scramble just to keep up.

Sheri talks about herself and feeling anxious when feeling rushed

I hardly am ever rushed by others. Being able to go at my own pace is awesome. When I'm not working I go at my own pace and don't have to answer to anyone or anything.

Now that I have a new dog I sometimes feel a self-imposed rushing to get everything done. This isn't a comfortable feeling. If I have a big list of things to do in a short amount of time then I'm in another frame of mind and no longer in that peaceful state. I'm feeling more anxious. On these days taking leisurely walks with my dog are out of the question and that's frustrating for me and him.

When I'm teaching I'm often rushing to get things done before the school kids come in the morning and it can be stressful. This is probably a common feeling for all of the teachers at the start of their day. Any kind of deadlines are like that I would imagine.

When we are patient with their muddling, dillydallying, and exasperation, we are showing trust in their ability to manage their lives.[22]

Author's reflections:
It is almost instinctive for us to want to save another person from embarrassment, failure or frustration. We cringe when they forget certain words or can't remember how to make tea and jump at the chance to make things right, whether they're having difficulty with something as simple as folding a towel or as difficult as giving a speech.

The big picture helps us remember that had we not gotten up each and every time we fell as a toddler we would not have developed the skills to walk. When we allow someone, even someone with great difficulties, to sometimes struggle for answers to their own problems, they learn important lessons. To have the patience to trust another's ability to grow through their efforts is to honor another person's dignity and pride of accomplishment.

What happens when you give the person you are caring for time to do things themselves?

Christie talks about giving her husband time to work things out

As a Caregiver I would often hover over my husband in my hyper-vigilance. Letting him figure things out on his own was difficult for me because I always wanted to help.

As far as Alzheimer's goes, I was told that I should try to keep my husband as relaxed as possible. This was tough in terms of knowing what he was still capable of and wanting him to be somewhat independent of my direction. I also needed to step in when he had lost certain skills. Over the seven years that he was home with me he went from splitting wood for the stove to picking up twigs for kindling. He went from doing the entire laundry to helping fold a few socks. I tried to help him feel good about his efforts, no matter what stage he was at. If I had lots of time I had no problem letting him try to figure things out but if I was rushed I wouldn't be so patient about his efforts and mistakes.

Sheri talks about teaching and allowing the time for her students to do their work

Life is good when I give others time for their projects. In the classroom, when you aren't rushing the children to do their work they are much happier. I give them time to explore and test the waters on their own.

Every single day I'm dealing with the idea of rhythm. If that's off then everything goes out of balance. Even if I stop to take a simple breath it helps to restore my natural flow. When my rhythm is in sync with my surroundings then it is easier for me to allow my students the time they need. When I'm feeling off then I have less patience and tend to want to hurry them.

Are you patient with the confusion and mistakes of the person you are caring for?

Christie talks about her patience with her husband's mistakes

Of course it depends on whether we were rushing to make a doctor's appointment, getting him to adult daycare, or getting me to work, whether I had the patience to handle his confusion. Those were the times that really tested me as a Caregiver. Most of the time I was fine and considered our life style challenging and on the edge.

Once in a while I wasn't up to it and I would watch as all my good intentions would crumble in a fit of rage. An example was the time he put the entire box of fabric softener sheets in the dryer. I couldn't believe it and got upset. Now it just seems funny. Then there was the time he put the tray for the wood burning stove in backwards so there was no handle to get it out. I was picturing having to replace the entire $2000 stove. Luckily I finally figured out a way to get it out. Again what seems funny now was very upsetting at the time and I wouldn't have considered myself as being patient with his mistakes.

Sheri talks about her partner and learning to be more patient

I'm getting much better at handling her struggles and confusion. She's the one I deal with this issue the most because she's the closest person to me. She can push my buttons because we are opposites so I feel like I've learned a lot in this area.

One thing I need to have patience for is how she has decided to take care of herself. For example when she takes her medicine on an empty stomach there's a good chance that she'll be ulcerating her stomach. When she does it she ends up in the bathroom vomiting. Even though she doesn't complain I can't ignore the things I see and hear. She knows these symptoms will happen but she doesn't change her behavior. It's hard for me to watch all this. I'm getting better and don't nag her about it like I used to. The problem is that it is affecting the quality of her life and the quality of our life together. If I wasn't around this behavior as much, or if it didn't affect the quality of my life

so much I probably wouldn't be so impatient or judgmental.
   I realized all of this was something in myself that I had to learn and that there was nothing wrong with her. It is easy for me to own my feelings now. Because she didn't shut down as we discussed our differences, I was able to learn these lessons and how to handle things. There was no discord. She was able to guide me in a nice way and that meant I didn't get all ruffled as we worked things out. I was able to grow.

Musings on Mayeroff:
Being patient involves being patient with ourselves as well. We need time to learn, grow, live and time to discover ourselves and the other person. Caring matures over time.[23]

Author's reflections:
In this world of instant success our ability to be patient with ourselves is being challenged in similar ways as our ability to be patient with others. Technology is a major contributor to the problem because it is all about faster and more. It encourages us to barely finish one task before going on to the next and then the next and again the next.
   Patience is about taking time for ourselves. The more time we take for ourselves, the more we learn about ourselves. Discovery and growth happen over long periods of time, and we have to have the patience to return to our life's lessons, to pick up where we left off. Lessons about our relationships, survival, fulfillment and purpose all need to be revisited from time to time. Sometimes we may have to repeat a lesson several times before it sinks in. Do we pick the right friends, are we doing work that is meaningful? Patience is necessary for all of this. The same kinds of lessons need to be learned in our Caregiving. Is this meaningful for us, are we doing a good job, how can we flourish within the challenges we face.

What happens when you take time to achieve insight into yourself and the person in your care?

Christie talks about taking the time to care for her husband and the growth it afforded both of them

Through the insights I gained while taking care of my husband I learned a lot about him and about this disease called Alzheimer's. There was still a piece of him that survived until his last day. His humor and his emotional connection were always there. I got to look closely at who he was and who he became as the disease progressed. There was plenty of time for this over the many years, months, days and hours we had together.
   I grew tremendously as I took time to care for my husband over the 8 years and later after taking more time to learn and grow from the experience. I don't think I knew how much the experience meant to me until a year after it was over. I can see now how I am more confident, more focused on my roles in life and more connected to the people I love.

Because I took that time for myself I feel like I can focus on what is truly important to me now. I can tell I'm different because when I see people having difficulties in their lives I have a sense now that there is always something deeper that holds things together in the end. Maybe it's love, connection, caring. I spend less time worrying about others or myself. Somehow I know we'll eventually make it through our momentary crisis until the day it all ultimately comes to an end. Until then I stay engaged and excited about this journey we all share.

Sheri talks about taking time for herself and time to learn about others

When I take the time for myself life gets better. It just keeps getting better. I love taking time to learn. That's why I became a teacher because I love to learn. It takes time to learn about others as well and I'm developing the patience for the journey of learning about others that life has taken me on.

Chapter 8

Seeing us both honestly

Musings on Mayeroff:
True caring comes about when we can honestly see the other person and are able to accept them as they truly are and not how we would prefer them to be.[24]

Author's reflections:
Unconditional love is something that we often aspire to but have difficulty achieving. Our brains act quickly to apply our lofty standards and ideals to our relationships. When we compare a loved one to others or set overly high expectations for ourselves and our relationship, the reality will most likely fall short of our imagined perfection.

When we can finally see the person we are caring for as they truly are and learn to love them "warts and all" we can then begin to properly care for them.

How do you juggle how the person you are caring for is today and how you would have preferred them to be?

Susan talks about her husband's recent disinterest in travel

We had always talked about traveling after retirement and now because of his illness my husband does not want to go anywhere anymore. I still had a desire to travel, even if it is on my own. I did struggle with this in the beginning of our journey into my husband's Alzheimer's. Of course if I had a magic wand I would have him change back to the guy who was going to be my traveling partner.

Since I'm a realistic sort of person I resolved my dilemma by having our friend stay with my husband. This freed me up to travel on my own to visit relatives or enjoy some of the places I've always wanted to visit. It isn't the same as sharing the experience with him but better than nothing. I can't say I want him to be any different because he has this disease and can't change that. Having Alzheimer's isn't the same as a personality quirk. I understand why he is so different now as part of his symptoms.

Barbara talks about how her husband truly was vs. how she would have liked him to be

I would have liked him to be more consistent with his health. In actuality he was doctor and medication dependent and he didn't think that any self-help like losing weight or taking care of himself in other ways would have any health benefits. He had all these specialists monitoring him every few months.

I wish he would have been more independently proactive and taken more responsibility for his health. Instead of being a passive spectator and depending on doctors to fix him, I would have preferred that he really understood self-care and things like nutrition. I wish he had made the connection that if he had lost weight he would have needed less medication. Lastly, he didn't believe in Internal Medicine but loved all the different specialists he went to. A generalist probably would have been the only kind of doctor who would have had the ability to find his cancer. No specialist was in charge of that part of his body so they didn't catch what was happening.

Before his cancer diagnosis I had a very difficult time caring for him and basically left it all up to him. Since my preferences for him were almost opposite to who he was I had to step back from his care. Once he was diagnosed all that changed. Both of us immediately understood how important it was for him to get the right care and that we would have to be a team for him to have a chance at survival.

Musings on Mayeroff:
As a Caregiver we must be able to look deeply and honestly into ourselves; this includes making sure that what we are doing for another is actually benefitting them. Is it helping them to grow or is it actually getting in their way?[25]

Author's reflections:
Being able to see ourselves honestly includes being able to see ourselves as Caregivers. Sometimes fear of not doing a good job prevents us from taking a true inventory of our caring. We want so much to think that we are doing things right that we "forget" to take stock. Approaching the caring relationship with self-awareness, courage and humility allows us to better assess our efforts and give an honest evaluation of our caring.

Do you evaluate your caring to see what is working?

Susan talks about evaluating her caring for her husband

I am constantly evaluating our situation to see what is working and what needs "tweaking". My husband's Alzheimer's has caused him to be an open book. He no longer has the ability to hide or fake anything due to the nature of his illness. It is easy for me to get good feedback about my care. His expressions are clear indications of what I am doing right and what might be upsetting to him. When I see him starting to get upset as quickly as I can I change the situation to help things go more smoothly for us both.

Barbara talks about evaluating her caring for her husband

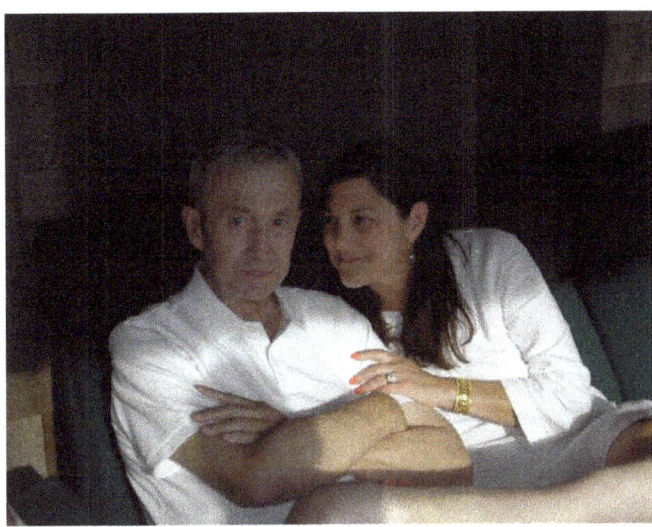

Barbara and her husband

At first nothing was going right in my Caregiving. This was before my husband found out about his cancer. I would state my case and then step back and watch my husband take things into his own hands. We had heated arguments about all of this. I could only go so far in making any demands or drawing a line in the sand. I had to say things like, "There's nothing I can do here if you don't take the necessary steps towards becoming more healthy." Then I would watch him making his own mistakes.

Once he was diagnosed with cancer things changed. He became more resigned to the path that he had chosen with his health. He had picked a certain way to live and was accepting of the results as they played out including that he had "drawn the short straw". He was never bitter about his destiny as it played out. The entire family held the belief that he had been completely himself throughout and had made his own choices.

As for my part there was no blame. I totally supported him and never used "I told you so" against him. This is when the real Caregiving began for me. I was able to evaluate my way of being with him and become part of his healthcare team. I accepted who he was and decided that it was more important for all of us to now work towards the same goal of his survival. Instead of fighting we worked together to find solutions to what was happening to him and we all hoped for the best outcome.

Musings on Mayeroff:
As a Caregiver we need to check in on ourselves from time to time to make sure we are motivated by a true desire to help another person. It is important to keep in mind that no one is perfect in their care and mistakes can be made. We must be able to admit our mistakes and be open to suggestions for improvement, for this is a part of being honest.[26]

Author's reflections:
Admitting to our mistakes sounds easy enough, but the actual act can be emotionally challenging.

When businesses make mistakes with their work or customer service they are usually able to keep their loyal customers by being honest in admitting they were wrong. When they fail to do this they may lose a customer or in the extreme, go out of business entirely. Politicians have the same option. When they admit their mistakes they appear more human and we are often able to forgive them. When their pride gets in the way or they blame others, the wise voter won't vote for them again.

When isolated Caregivers insist on gathering information on their own and refuse to take the support that is being offered by professionals, they run the risk of making mistakes in their Caregiving. Being open to the mentoring of experts and heeding their suggestions often helps a Caregiver to make good decisions. It is up to the Caregiver to admit that they have more of a chance to make mistakes when they insist on "going it alone." Being open to suggestions and support is part of honestly assessing their role and situation.

How do you handle your own mistakes?

Susan talks about how she handles mistakes with her husband

Sometimes I find myself having a discussion about something that my husband cannot understand. When I see that he is showing resistance because he can't grasp what I am saying I change my approach. First I realize that I need to correct the mistake in how I approached the topic by backing out of the conversation and agreeing with his view. Later I can start all over with a new approach to make things better.

Barbara talks about how she handled mistakes with her husband

I think I should have forced the issue and had him checked out by an Internal Medicine doctor. When he got sick with cancer, I felt like I had "allowed him" to not go and that could be considered a mistake on my part. It was my fatal error. Since his death I've been able to let myself off the hook about it. I did what I thought was right at the time.

Once the critical care started, there was nobody more on top of it than me. The research, the communication, the support, and the creating a world of buoyancy wasn't just about caring for his health. It was about honor; honoring him, myself and the situation. It has changed me forever.
Mistakes are no longer anything I fear because I can always correct something that goes wrong. I am able to come from this deep level of engagement as I live my life now.

Musings on Mayeroff:
Worrying more about what the neighbors will think about our

caring interferes with our ability to actually meet the needs of the person being cared for.[27]

Author's reflections:
In Caregiving the idea of "keeping up appearances" holds little water. When we are truly engaged in our caring we are searching for an intrinsic benefit for the person cared for and not the appearance of top-notch Caregiving to others.

Outsiders who don't know the whole situation are in no position to cast a judgmental eye in our direction. When we give others the right to judge us we hand them our power, and this hurts our caring.

If I allow myself to worry about what others think about my Caregiving, I am less able to be the strong, powerful advocate that I need to be for the person I am caring for.

What do you think about how others see your caring? Is their view helpful to seeing yourself honestly?

Susan talks about how others view her caring for her husband

Most people cannot understand how I can remain so positive. I'm positive because I know this is where my life has brought me. I believe that God will always be with me and help to carry all my burdens. I can just concentrate on the journey without worrying about what is coming next. I certainly don't worry about the judgments of others because I feel confident that I am doing a great job with my husband. Since I'm the one living this extraordinary experience I feel that I know myself more honestly than anyone who isn't with me all the time. It helps to be a very aware person, which I am.

Barbara talks about how others saw her caring for her husband

I have a style of caring now that is identified with me as others see me. There is dignity and honor to the way I care and people see that. Early on in my life I would base my day on helping others in my family to have a good day. Their happiness would represent a good day for me. Back then it wasn't really selfless on my part or truly about honoring another. I previously needed to have control in that kind of caring.

As a Caregiver for my husband I had to tap into my selflessness. Others saw me as drawn to the role of Caregiver in almost a chemical attraction sort of way. I agreed and saw it as a continuum of the relationship I had always had with my husband.

I've never said this out loud before but after my husband died I felt a bit like I was losing a type of celebrity. While I was caring for him the entire town would ask about how he was doing and how I was handling it. His brothers called me on his first birthday after his passing, which was only three weeks later, to comfort me. A year later there is none of that.

In the work I do now, I support families going through similar issues and it feels like I have re-entered the world of Caregiving again. When I accomplish things for my clients and cut through the obstacles along their path I enjoy the effects I am having on improving their lives. Their appreciation helps me to see myself more honestly as a person with an extraordinary ability to continually care deeply for others.

Author's reflections:
When we put someone up on a pedestal we make it impossible for us to care for them. We need to be able to see them honestly to know what they truly need to get through the day or overcome great obstacles. Having rigid ideas about them, whether negative or positive, does not allow them to grow and change for the better.
  Our judgments and opinions can get in the way of seeing the other person honestly. If we think our opinion about them is correct then we are no longer looking for the truth in the situation. In effect we are not allowing our own selves to grow if we become overly defensive about our care.
  Another thing that limits our ability to know another is when we rush to get things done quickly or more easily. In not being willing to take the time, we prevent the other from growing based on their trial and error. We instead narrow the picture of that person's experience and strengths and inhibit their own successes and failures.
  Jumping to the end game of what we want for the other prevents us from sharing in the unfolding of their path towards self-knowledge. A diploma doesn't substitute for the years of study, nor does a trophy substitute for the excitement of preparing for the game. Being in the moment and seeing the other person honestly allows them to both stumble and shine as their path unfolds. We get to learn about them through these struggles, successes and failures.
  Some of us will be Caregivers for people we haven't known for very long. As we get to know them better, it is helpful to be mindful of the sincerity of the growing relationship. When either of us shows a false face to the other, we weaken the fiber of that growing trust.
  When caring for people we have known a long time, maybe even our whole lives, it's even harder to hide our true selves. Our parents, spouse or children can usually "read" us in how we speak or in our body language. If what they find is our restlessness, irritability or fear, instead of growing closer they may pull away. We, of course, may feel unappreciated, resentful, or even feel as if we should give up when we are not being seen for who we truly are.

Musing on Mayeroff:
Honesty is woven into the fabric of caring.[28]

Author's reflections:
To be a successful Caregiver it is important to spend a good deal of our Caregiving time observing the other person's ways while being honest with ourselves about our feelings and expectations in this relationship. Honesty sets the stage for taking the high road when we are caring for another person.

There are many things that get in the way of getting to know both the person we are caring for as well as ourselves. These are but a few: needing to be right, skipping the day to day feelings to focus on the final outcome, expediency, worship, having a split between our actions and feelings, and pretending to be or feel differently. Are there any examples that you can think of where you exhibited one of these traits?

Susan talks about behaving honestly with her husband

I have never had a problem in this area as I was raised to be honest and realistic about life. I carry this over into my caring for my husband. I don't need to be right. I'm always looking for ways to do things better and am open to new ideas. I enjoy the day to day caring and don't focus on where this all will lead. I don't put my husband up on a pedestal. I feel that I am being myself and don't need to pretend to be someone else.

Barbara talks about her husband

I felt that I needed to be right when it came to my husband's health insurance. There was a time before we had children when he didn't believe in health insurance. When he left his corporate job he just didn't think health insurance was necessary and that it was a waste of money.

I completely disagreed. I had health insurance through my job. I've never been without health insurance for my entire life. We weren't married yet so I couldn't put him on my policy. This would be entirely his expense. I didn't understand how he could ignore the risk he was taking and not be covered for any eventuality. I wondered that if our priorities were so different would we be able to work this out. I wasn't particularly interested in knowing this side of him or accepting it. I was convinced I was right.

He was under the gun because in twenty four months he would have had to start all over with health insurance as though he had never had it so pre-existing conditions and other limitations would have kicked in.

I finally convinced him to buy the insurance before time ran out and when you talk about expediency I remember even paying for it for a short time. My split between my actions and my feelings was that I felt that I needed to step in on this issue because I was convinced that he needed health insurance so badly. My real feelings were that I would have preferred it if he had taken the lead on this and bought his own but that honestly wasn't who he was.

Chapter 9
The courage of trust

Musings on Mayeroff:
Because we cannot know the outcome when we trust another person to follow his or her own path in life, we need to be prepared to tackle the unpredictable future.[29]

Author's reflection:
When it comes to illness, the worst thing that most of us would want to hear is, "We don't know what you have and we don't know how to treat it." As painful as it is to hear the news that a loved one has diabetes, Alzheimer's disease, or cancer, it is also easier to hear. Surprisingly most of us prefer the certainty of a firm diagnosis over the confusion of not knowing what the heck is going on.

In Caregiving for the sick, we often don't have certainty or answers to the many questions surrounding the disease's progression—or even diagnosis on occasion--our patient's ability to adjust to their condition as they struggle down their path, how involved we need to become, and many other unknowns, and it is unsettling. As Caregivers, we need to expect the unexpected and to trust in ourselves that we can be of support in helping the person we are caring for meet those boat-rocking eventualities. It takes courage to accomplish this.

How does it affect your caring not to know where your loved one's path will lead?

Suzanne talks about her husband's last five months

My husband and I were both always optimistic people. Our outlook was that we trusted that the best outcome would happen for us. That's why it was a shock when we learned that he was back in the intensive care unit. We weren't expecting a negative outcome.

After his heart surgery in November, until his death in April, my daughter and I were there for him in whatever he needed. He trusted completely that we would be there for him and we trusted ourselves that we could give him that.

He was in and out of the hospital during this entire time and until his last day we remained optimistic and trusted for the best. My attitude was that I trusted that he would get through it. That was his attitude also. Because he was so certain of his recovery he even encouraged me to put rental money down on a house in Florida for the winter so we would have something to look forward to. That could be considered the evidence of how trusting

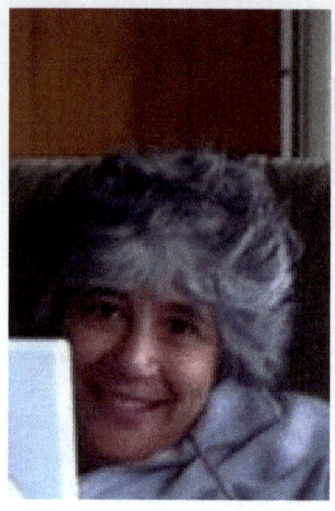
Toni

we were that things would go well. Even though we had no idea that he was near the end of his life we always trusted that he would make it. Of course no one can know the future but we had our strong belief to keep us going.

Toni talks about her mother having early onset Alzheimer's disease before anyone knew much about it

No one in my family had any idea of where this disease would take all of us. 25 years ago there was very little information about early onset Alzheimer's and no one was really speaking about it. It was a new diagnosis, and for a long time they didn't know what she had.

My father and I had the attitude that we would do everything that we could for her, and in the end we trusted that somehow we would conquer the disease. We would change her diet or try anything new that we heard about for Alzheimer's. Of course we couldn't know how things would ultimately turn out but we naively thought that there was nothing that we couldn't conquer. Some of this was our denial and some of this was our strong trust in our ability to care and the hope that that would be enough to save her in the end.

I tried to be right there in the moment to see what she needed for the most comfortable life possible. I trusted that she would flourish as much as she was able with this kind of care and I always tried to have her self-esteem stay strong. Just like she made me feel good about myself I wanted to give that to her regardless of where any of this was taking us. I trusted that this was what she needed and I had no doubts that I could do this for her.

Author's reflections:
Trusting another person doesn't come easily, partly because we can't know the other's soul or their intentions. For mutual trust to last, both parties should be able to deal with the unexpected, which is sure to arise. It is impossible to ever be 100% certain of anything, but our trust helps us to believe and hope in the other. In an ideal caring relationship trust includes setting the stage for a favorable outcome where trust can flourish.

There are many things that get in the way of trust. One of the main difficulties with trusting another is that personal histories get in the way. Some people who don't trust have had serious earlier experiences of that trust being betrayed. They shut down, often, for fear of being too open to being let down. Others can't handle the unknowable aspect of trust and instead insist on guarantees for how it will all turn out. They become overly protective, controlling and distrustful towards others. An example would be a Caregiver who refuses to trust a doctor unless they guarantee that they can cure the person they are caring for. Instead of trust they challenge every recommendation or suggestion or jump from doctor to doctor until someone makes the guarantees they need to hear.

Insisting on guarantees and being overly protective are two ways to destroy trust and there are several others. If someone cares too much trust can change into obsession. In some institutionalized religions this is encouraged. The authority figures would rather foster blind trust from their congregation. In this case the authority is not trusting that "their flock" will eventually come to their own morally sound conclusions.

Another way of viewing the world that interferes with trust is the need to have unwavering opinions about things. We often come across people preoccupied with being right all the time. This negates self-trust which implies an ability to be comfortable with yourself and with not being able to know everything. Ideally you are trusting yourself to find good answers to life's questions. In contrast having to be right focuses attention on just that need to be right and inspires indifference towards learning from others, leaving no opening for trust of self or others.

What stories come to mind with the words trust, independence, overprotection, needing to be right, preparing the environment for success?

Suzanne talks about trust and preparing the environment for her husband

We trusted each other but over the years I became overly protective of my husband in all sorts of situations, not only his healthcare. Because he trusted me he would listen to what I had to say.

During our marriage he gave me a great deal of independence and trusted my potential to take on more challenges in my life. He also encouraged me to go back and get my Master's at the age of 50. He encouraged me to become involved in many organizations like Inner Wheel, which is an offshoot of Rotary. He also encouraged me to travel and be independent. Other friends of mine had husbands who were more restrictive about their activities but my husband was never that way.

While I was caring for my husband I don't know if I needed to be right or wasn't trusting others to do their jobs but I had a very bad temper and could fly off the handle. It seemed I was easily excitable. I think that the stress of years and years of being hyper vigilant took its toll. Either I'm now mellowing, or since he passed I'm calmer now. I don't really know what I would attribute that to. Maybe now that I'm not a Caregiver anymore I can finally relax.

In terms of preparing the environment for success, I did the bulk of the driving when we went to medical appointments together. That way he could rest. I also was the homemaker. Those were ways I could support him and his recovery from his health issues.

Toni talks about being overprotective with her mother

Overprotection and preparing the environment for success come to mind out of that group of words. My overprotection did come out of my not trusting that things would work themselves out. Because we were dealing with Alzheimer's I felt I needed to be more involved in my mother's care. I was always trying to make the environment comfortable for her during her early onset Alzheimer's.

The following are some examples of my being overly protective. Since she wasn't doing much initiating anymore, it was up to me to make sure she got out and experienced the world everyday. When we went to restaurants I made sure she would have loads of napkins so that the second she spilled something I would clean it up. That way she could feel that she was just like everybody else. In terms of eating I made sure there were finger foods and things that were easy to manage. I checked her body functions to make sure everything was regulated properly. I sort of feel with Alzheimer's that this degree of care is needed and that trusting the person themselves to do all this wasn't realistic anymore.

In terms of setting up the environment for success I would observe her difficulties and try to solve any problems. I trusted that if I did this well she would flourish as much as she was able to. If she started spilling a drink I would put liquids in a child's sippy cup to help her successfully drink. Once she could no longer use a spoon or a knife we cut things or had her use a fork. I did all the research to find tools to help her be independent for as long as possible. I never put her down ever for anything and always acted as if she had expressed herself clearly. We set her up for a very pleasant life as much as possible.

When she needed monitoring, my dad and I set it up so that she could be observed, safe and independent at the same time without being aware of the monitoring. This made sure that she didn't get lost, and we also had her wear identification once her language skills started to lapse. We tried to keep her life as normal as possible.

Musings on Mayeroff:

Trust in one's own ability to grow is needed before we are able to trust another's path towards growth. If we are only trying to fit ourselves into an overused and outgrown mold, with no room to expand, it is unlikely that we would want more than that for another.[30]

Author's reflections:
Our own limitations become the limitations we impose on others. If I can't even conceive of exceeding what has always been expected of me, it will be hard for me to accept another's evolution beyond that. As we trust our own ability to change, we become able to feel more and more excited for others as they flourish. Trust that we can grow, learn and create is at the root of our development and is needed so that we can trust in the growth of another.

Our ability to change affects our caring. Do you feel that you were able to trust that you would grow during your Caregiving experience?

Toni talks about growing while she cared for her mother

I'm not sure I was aware of the trust I had in myself at the time to grow but I was living the truth of that trust. There was no question that I, as a daughter, would be there to care for my mom. It was certainly expected of me by my family. I trusted this too and never questioned that it couldn't be done or shouldn't be done.

Beyond the trust of my just being there was my growth into an extremely patient and unbelievably loving person. As I said I may not have been aware of the trust that I could do this at the time but I embraced the changes in myself. I grew past the idea of having a mother to care for me to the idea that we were all a family and I needed to care for her safety and dignity as a member of our family.

Musings on Mayeroff:
Trusting someone else's process involves trusting my ability to care as they become involved in their struggle. When I care like this, I also need to be confident that I can learn from and correct my own mistakes. Trusting my instincts is a significant part of this confidence.[31]

Author's reflections:
In Caregiving I am partaking in another's journey. I may at one time be keenly intuitive and aligned with their path, and at other times I may stray. My confidence comes from being able to pick myself up and correct my mistakes as best I can. I can then use my intuition wisely and begin to trust those "gut feelings" we all get in the midst of an experience, or when reflecting about how best to proceed. I can act on these on-target gut feelings, and use their applications in my Caregiving, enhancing the experience.

How does your trust in your ability to learn from your mistakes, make good judgments and rely on your instincts play out in your Caregiving?

Suzanne talks about trusting herself as she cared for her husband

I don't think I made any mistakes except for the fact that I was too reliant on doctors. I was too trusting of them and didn't question their decisions. There was a steep learning curve for me and it wasn't until a week before my husband passed away that I ever spoke up to a doctor. I had doctors in my family and thought of them almost like a god. It was hard to trust myself because this was a shock to find that a doctor would be so reckless.

Even though my husband had a small stroke after an angiogram in the fall and it turns out his heart blockage was only 30% in one artery, they still decided to do the bypass surgery that ultimately killed him. I didn't see the results of the tests until it was too late. When I did I was furious and trusted my gut feeling enough to finally speak up. When I saw the doctor coming down the hall to see my husband I told him I wouldn't allow him in the room. That's how upset I was. I've never spoken up to any other doctor like that.

Otherwise, generally I trusted myself that I was making good judgments along the way as I gathered information. I felt that I could trust my instincts. We also had our daughter to bounce ideas off of. She was very close to her father. She didn't really offer opinions but she was there to listen to both of us as we struggled to get information and make good decisions.

Toni talks about her view about making mistakes with her mother

It was explained to me that if I make a mistake I shouldn't beat myself up for it. I learned to trust myself from my dad. He would tell me to be your own best friend and trust your instincts. Hindsight is 20/20 and with the information I had, I have to trust that I did the best that I could for my mother and later my brother.

After my dad passed, when I would make mistakes, I would remember his lessons. I would tell myself that I had done the best with what I knew and to trust this. After I took over being my mother's primary Caregiver I often didn't have all the information I needed to make good decisions. I didn't feel guilty about my mistakes because my intention was always to surround her with love and make her life as comfortable as possible. Once she went into the nursing home this wasn't always possible. It wasn't only up to me anymore.

I learned a lot from caring for my mother. It was a loving beyond loving. She had always taught me to balance independence with interdependence and now I was learning to relate to her intuitively in the same way. Even when she eventually ended up rocking back and forth in a chair I didn't want her to feel like a child. I used my intuitive powers to connect to her in any way I could think of and carefully watched her reactions to things I would do or say. She wasn't a child. She was my mother even though her skills had diminished. She was still an important person to me, a person I loved and would do anything for.

Chapter 10

The humility in learning

Musings on Mayeroff:
Humility is the ability to humble ourselves or become deferential to others, putting our own needs and opinions on an equal or even lower footing than theirs.

When we face new and challenging circumstances with humility, we are better equipped to confront them with a broad perspective. When humble, we're also likely to step back, evaluate a situation, and resume in a better light. Humility helps us to bypass our ego when dealing with difficult situations as well. We have less "invested" in the old ways of problem solving and possible damage to our pride. Humility helps us explore new avenues to resolution.[32]

Author's reflections:
There is humility in thinking that there is always more to learn. The world is full of lessons and sometimes these lessons show up in the most unlikely places. We can learn about caring from others who are walking down similar paths, and we can also learn from those whose experiences are very different from ours.

When we strive to make our caring better, we learn about ourselves, our potential for creativity, our boundaries, our feelings and much more. Even our mistakes have lessons to offer us when evaluated in humility.

When we hold on to the belief that we "know it all" we run the risk of becoming stagnant and uninspired in our caring. We see others as only being there to satisfy our needs but not as a source for our learning. No one gets to blossom if we stay locked in our old ways.

If we approach life as a learning and growing process, we'll experience the world filling us with curiosity and vitality. Searching for the solution to various problems challenges us to reach deeper into ourselves and discover the resources that are within as well as all around us.

Successful and unsuccessful caring happens in all sorts of situations. What happens when someone isn't truly caring or humble in a work setting? Do you know of times where a boss or authority figure didn't actually care for their employees and because of their ego acted as if they had nothing further to learn from their interactions with them?

Patrice talks about projects she has worked on

I have worked with "leaders" that seem to think leading means dictating. They seem more arrogant than humble and didn't know how to partner with others. In those situations very little learning goes on for them.

In contrast good leading is a give and take. I use this principal when I care for my autistic son. I have also experienced this good kind of caring in my work situation. The best boss I have ever had was more humble and made me feel like I worked with her not for her. Throughout my career I have found ways to work with her again and again because of her leadership style.

Joe M. talks about other business owners he's heard about and about himself as an employer

I've heard of situations that weren't directly related to me, where the employers didn't take care of their employees. They think of each one of them as just a number that punches a clock. There's just no relationship with the employees as to how or what they are doing in their lives outside of work and no willingness to learn either.

When a boss treats his employees like that he simply doesn't have long term employees. In some cases their egos as employers seem to crush their own human feelings. They end up satisfying their huge egos more than even their business needs. Over the years I've noticed that these ego problems occur more frequently at the level of middle management because most business owners understand that happy employees are better for the success of their business.

Since I've always owned my own business I've been in the position of being the boss. Just as I found it important to care for my wife when she became ill, I have also found it important to care for my employees over the years when they have faced difficult circumstances. I've taken an interest in their problems and tried to find ways to help them solve them. Sometimes this meant looking outside the box for resources or solutions to help them. When I made mistakes I learned from them. My pride had nothing to do with it. When a crisis would arise for an employee all I cared about was how could I make this situation better for them.

Musings on Mayeroff:

The humility that we bring to our Caregiving can act as a mirror into ourselves. If, by being humble, we show others that we neither aggrandize nor try to conceal our true selves, we can also allow them to see our vulnerability.[33]

Author's reflections:
Caring with humility allows a Caregiver the chance to share with others the many facets of their character. Being humble allows us to be open about ourselves, our foibles and failings. It allows those around us to come to know us more completely.

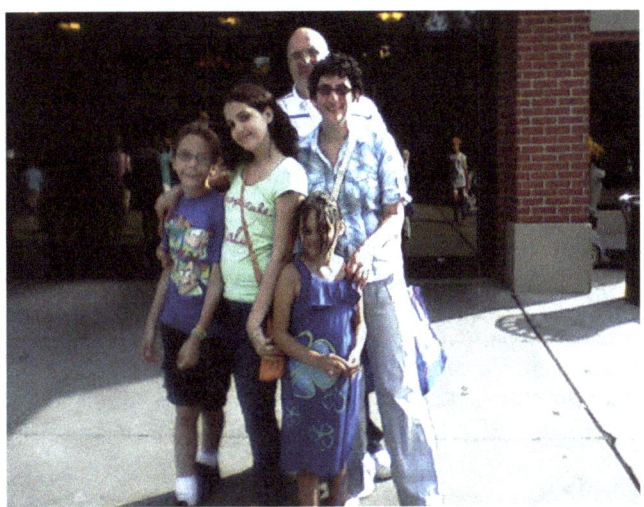

Patrice and family

    Instead of sharing their true feelings with others, sometimes Caregivers would rather defensively shield themselves from the toll Caregiving is taking on them or the lack of support they are feeling. Instead of asking for help or sharing how they are really feeling they take more and more control over the situation in an attempt to mold it to their needs. Rather than humility, a Caregiver can start to demonstrate an exaggerated view of him or herself. They may begin to seem detached and have a "go it alone" attitude, masking the sense of vulnerability that lies beneath the surface. All they are willing to share with the very support network that might be of assistance to them are the responses of either "I'm fine." or "No, I don't need anything." Those that work in the field of Family Caregiving have heard these phrases over and over.

Do you know anyone who is a Caregiver who has ignored their need for help from others, making instead a show of their perceived strength?

Patrice talks about going it alone when caring for her son

As a parent of a child on the autistic spectrum, my main goal as a Caregiver is to make my son as independent as possible. When my husband is at work and I'm on my own, there are times that I am just trying to get through the day, especially when my son is struggling. Then instead of being a Caregiver I go into survival mode. In the middle of those times I forget to ask for help. Being on my own during the day causes me to sometimes forget that I can make those struggles teachable moments too as much as possible. It shows me that I need to have more help to be able to stay at the level of Caregiving that makes me feel that I am doing a good job. I have a big family and sometimes it's just a matter of asking so I can take a break.

Musings on Mayeroff:
When we look over our shoulder at other Caregiving relationships, to see whose burden is greater, or whose care is more generous, we are taking time away from attending to the wellbeing of the one we are caring for.[34]

Author's reflections:
We all do it. We wonder what it would be like to walk in another person's shoes. Caregivers especially wonder. They wonder if taking care of someone with mental illness is more difficult than their job of caring for someone with dementia. Is it more challenging to care for someone who spends most of their day in a wheelchair or to care for a hyperactive child with autism? The comparisons are numerous and ultimately a waste of the Caregiver's time.

Musings on Mayeroff:
When we admit that there is much we don't know and are open to learn more, we are showing our humility. We can always learn more about how best to care for another and about the person we care for. This learning can come from closely monitoring our interaction with our loved one and their behavior through conversation or observation.[35]

Author's reflection:
It is said that when a martial artist first receives their black belt that along with the belt comes the realization of how much more there is to learn. Caregiving is such a complex task that, for a Caregiver who shows humility and other positive traits, there is no end to the learning. There are the medical terms, the legal and financial decisions, the emotional ups and downs. Then there are the changing lifestyles and relationships that intersect with that of the Caregiver and the person they are caring for. Humility and a desire to learn keep Caregivers on track and honest about the fact that there is still more to discover.

Have you known people who are humble and always curious and learning? Give any examples you can think of. How can this apply to learning in Caregiving?

Patrice talks about her humbleness in learning from her son

I use Mother Teresa as an example of humility. For this generation she was the ultimate Caregiver, sacrificing everything and always keeping a smile on her face. All her quotes point to the concept that caring for others is something that when you do it, you gain from it.

For me, staying humble often means trying to keep myself out of it altogether. To care for my son since his communication skills still get jumbled means I often have to try to get into his head as much as possible. I have to put the way I look at the world aside and think about how he is looking at it. When I can discover how he is seeing the situation I can figure out how to teach him to navigate the world as others might. I try to respect the way he looks at things and at the same time am able to show him how to look at it in another way.

Joe M. talks about his children being life-long learners

I think my children learned a lot from the experience of caring for their mother. As younger children they also learned directly from her because she was a caring person and in the role as their mother taught them to be the same way. For their entire lives they've continued to be humble and caring for their families and friends and probably for people they don't even know.

They learned this caring from both of us but their mother was the type of person who could talk to someone that she didn't even know in the supermarket for ten minutes. You just had to watch her in action and the lessons of caring were there. She was a great role model for our kids.

Chapter 11
Building on our strengths, recognizing our weaknesses

Musings on Mayeroff:
Our strengths can make us proud and our limitations can give us the space for humility and the search for additional resourcefulness.[36]

Author's reflections: Living a life based on the best use of our strengths helps to make us happy. Acknowledging our strengths with humility makes us proud that we are living a life based on the best we have to offer. In contrast, when we recognize our limitations, we can use our inner resources to overcome them. If we are open about our shortcomings, we can allow others to support us in our efforts in overcoming them. We all have both strengths and limitations and we enrich our lives when we strive to make use of our strengths over our weaknesses.

It's easy to be troubled by what we perceive to be our weaknesses and/or inadequacies. Have you experienced this in your Caregiving? How?

Sarah talks about the feelings of inadequacy in herself and her support groups

With my mother's cancer and with the Caregivers in my *Caring for Someone with Cancer* support groups, the theme of the inevitability of the progression of the illness, and the fact that there is nothing we can do as Caregivers to intervene, causes tremendous amounts of guilt. This occurs even though our logic says it is irrational to think we can cure our loved ones. It is definitely a perceived inadequacy. There is a powerlessness in the fact that we can't turn the disease around.

The members of the group also have a lot of guilt around doing something for themselves, even coming to the support group. They feel that needing a break is a weakness and they should be home, doing more for their partner. The guilt is also however quickly followed by anger at the situation they are in. They feel trapped and resentful.

Some Caregivers came to the group early in the diagnosis and they expressed their feelings of inadequacy about what to do, how long their caring would go on and what to expect. Examples were that they wondered if they should still work or go to all the medical appointments or should they be more separate. Just not knowing everything there was to know about Caregiving was perceived as a weakness.

Sarah talks about experiencing what she considered her weaknesses with her mother

When my mother was diagnosed twice with cancer it was hard for her to really believe it because she didn't feel sick at all. She refused treatments and lived for 14 months during which I was her main Caregiver. At a certain point she fell and broke her arm which may have been a sign of the spread of the cancer.

During this time I never felt confident that I was doing a good enough job caring for her and as a result I felt bad about needing a vacation. I made all her medical appointments and went with her. I did her laundry and cooked for her and even though I wasn't living with her I experienced anxiety each time the phone rang. She finally needed someone to live with her after her fall but even though we found someone to stay with her, I still felt conflicted about taking a vacation.

In this case I was the one who thought it was a weakness on my part to need a break from Caregiving. Because I felt guilty about leaving I realized I still wanted my mother's love and acknowledgement and wasn't getting it. I almost needed her approval to leave. Her disease caused her to be more self-involved so it was hard for her to appreciate what I was doing for her. Because she wasn't helping me to feel like I was doing a good job I now think that it would have been up to me to develop the confidence to leave for a short break. I shouldn't have waited for a sign of her appreciation to know that I was doing a good job for her and deserved a break.

Christie talks about her weaknesses in her caring for her husband

It's all about what I remember first, my kindness or my anger and frustration. Usually the times I lost my temper with my husband or experienced frustration or couldn't solve a problem come to mind without much effort. I feel awful when I think about them. Like the time I took him over to the local nursing home and told him if he didn't stop acting crazy in the car I'd just drop him off over there. Or the time I was yelling so loudly I was sure Adult Protective Services would send someone over to our house. I felt that my lack of patience was a weakness in me.

The thousands upon thousands of times that I was kind, patient, creative, funny and went out of my way to do something I knew he would enjoy take much more effort to conjure up. I was able to take him on family trips to California. We often went to movies that I picked because I knew he would be able to follow the story or enjoy the visuals. All at great effort on my part, planning, packing, anticipating....

I even had him training for athletic events and competing well into his Alzheimer's. Again the logistics of this were complex and required lots of extra effort on my part to make sure we were both fed, hydrated, equipped, properly dressed etc. This level of organization is difficult even for one athlete, never mind for the two of us. I suppose the fact that I never asked for help was an inadequacy, but at the time I felt that needing help would have been the weakness on my part.

I often wonder why it is easier for me to remember my inadequacies, my bad moods, fatigue, stress and failures as a Caregiver. It is a mystery but I've seen other Caregivers follow the same logic, so I know I'm not the only one who has this lopsided perspective.

Musings on Mayeroff:
The challenges that come along with caring hold a mirror up to this portrait of ourselves, one that shows our unique combination of strengths and weaknesses.[37]

Author's reflections:
Caregiving is often considered a test. Non-Caregivers may observe Caregivers and wonder if they themselves could ever measure up in the same way. We are being tested to the very essence of who we are as people, lovers, friends, family, attendants, servants and advocates. As we respond to the various demands that come up, we get to see exactly what cloth we are cut from. No two Caregivers are the same, nor are two situations exactly alike in the Caregiving world.

Caregiving is a test of our strengths. Name some of the strengths you have either discovered or put to use during your Caregiving. How did you utilize them?

Sarah talks about her strengths in her caring for her mother

One of my strengths is being able to find the necessary resources because I am very organized. This helped with being able to talk to doctors and get the information we needed. Because I was organized I was also able to plan day trips and bring happiness into my mother's life by taking her places that I knew she would enjoy. I provided an appealing alternative to the medical difficulties she was facing.

Another strength that I learned I had was my being able to still be compassionate towards a person like my mother where there had been a history of conflict and struggle. I was able to put that aside and not abandon her when she needed me. I feel this is one of my strengths, the ability to still be kind in spite of our history.

Sarah talks about the strengths of a woman in her Caregiver's support group

A woman in the support group's strengths was her creativity and persistence. She was able to organize a fund raiser for her loved one to have reconstructive surgery after her double mastectomy. It was a very clever and caring idea and the event was quite successful. I had never heard of anything being done like that before.

When I was running the support groups I developed a lot of respect and appreciation for what these Caregivers were able to do, how good they were at it and how they were able to keep their emotions stable for the most part. I often praised them for their strengths and the good job they were doing because most of them had no real objective awareness of what it was they were doing. Time for self reflection is scarce in many Caregiving situations.

Christie talks about her strengths in caring for her husband

I've had lots of training and experience as a teacher. My training turned out to be a strength for me. It has allowed me to understand that everyone learns differently, that tasks need to be broken down into their components, that organization and planning help things go more smoothly. All of this awareness that I acquired as a teacher came in handy during the time I cared for my husband.

Alzheimer's disease isn't just one symptom of memory loss and it certainly doesn't follow a stable, predictable progression. From minute to minute my husband would need help in many different areas, at levels of his ability that would change over time, and I had the complicated task of understanding where he was at and what he could handle.

One of my strengths was that I could tell almost intuitively what he would be able to do. I was able to design tasks for him at his level of skill. For example, he was always involved in the laundry over the years but his jobs went from doing the whole wash to finally just being able to transport the clothes upstairs for me to fold. Of course there were many stages in between. Over the seven years in the garden he went from complex pruning to picking up twigs for kindling. I was always vigilant about assessing when it was time to simplify a role. As a teacher it was usually easy for me to see the changes as they occurred. I did miss some of his changes for short periods. This was part of my denial when I realized I would then have to take over the lost skill myself. More work for me, arrrgh!

Another strength I have is being an optimistic problem solver. When things would start changing for the worse with my husband I would think of what I should do next as a question that had an answer, even though I couldn't always find the answer right away.

The driving situation became difficult after about four years. He would get anxious in the car and ask a bunch of questions. I considered this one of my greatest challenges but I, in my optimism, always believed that there would be an answer.

I was always trying new things to distract him and help us arrive safely. We performed David Mamet type plays with me improvising around his questions and short statements. I would introduce foreign accents to get him off a topic when explanations failed to calm him. I would get him to answer his own questions. His favorite music often helped and we would sing as we drove down the highway together. I would have "time outs" and pull off the highway and park for a time until things calmed down. All of these solutions to problems worked for a time until I needed to find something else that worked.

Someone once said I have an agile brain, another strength, and thankfully it came in handy with my problem solving abilities. I think if I had been more of a pessimist I wouldn't have been as creative or resourceful in finding solutions.

Another strength I had was the idea that we were separate people with different needs. I knew that at other times in my life I had become burnt out from giving too much of myself without replenishing my stores of patience, energy and quiet time.

Right from the beginning of my husband's Alzheimer's I made sure that I would keep as much of my life and schedule intact as I was able. Of course this became much more difficult towards the later years but I was determined. I still competed at a high level as an elite strength and endurance athlete, which required many months of training each year. My solution to caring for him at the same time was to bring him with me to the gym, or on my runs, and I even had him join in the competition for as long as he was able. I did the same thing as I switched to my annual triathlon competitions. He would bike, run and swim with me and then I had someone stay with him in the audience while I competed. Since this was in the later stages, the arrangements were more complicated, but I still had to try to live my life and not have both of us swallowed up into his disease.

Even though he was losing much of his musical ability, I had my music to keep me involved in my own life. I knew I needed to keep my skills up for my sanity to continue. I took my husband to lessons, to jam sessions, to gigs. He would scat sing in the workshops and jam sessions and again I was able to hire someone to care for him in the audience at my gigs. My strength was knowing what I needed and at the same time caring for him. I understand now that I needed good boundaries and a strong will to keep the things I loved in my life.

Continuing to work was difficult. As my humility grew and I started admitting that I needed help and asking for it, I found Adult Day Care centers that took care of my husband as I spent a few hours in my office. On other days I would bring him to the office and set up a treatment room with a DVD player, lunch and the birds while I would treat my acupuncture clients next door in another treatment room. All of this was designed to give me the feeling that my life was important too and nourished my caring efforts for the long haul of the eight years that my husband needed me.

Musings on Mayeroff:
Our pride recognizes clearly our accomplishments as they are tied to our strengths and limitations. We know what our strengths are, how we have known to ask for and accept outside support and how we have understood our dependency on various conditions.[38]

Author's reflections:
False pride originates in our insecurities and a denial of our limitations. We want to make ourselves and others feel good about what we are doing but we not willing to own up to the truth of who we really are and the situations that we find ourselves in. As a result there is an incorrect appraisal of what our strengths, limitations and situations are.

True pride comes from reflecting on a life that flows honestly from our strengths, limitations and good intentions. It is a humble pride that includes appreciation for the people and situations that helped us to be our best.

Have you been able to be proud of your strengths and appreciative of various conditions that have helped you?

Sarah talks about her pride in taking care of her mom

I was proud of the things I was good at in taking care of my mother. This helped me to not feel guilty after she died. I was really, really glad about that because it saved me from second guessing myself or going over and over my doubts.

I felt like I did what I could for her. Things like spending an entire day on the phone with Sloan Kettering to find the right person to go to for a second opinion, and after 40 calls finally being successful. She would not have done that for herself. She would have just dropped it. I am proud of my persistence and happy about my being so responsible in my caring.

One condition that I had to deal with was not helpful. I found that the progression of the cancer was always ahead of my efforts. For example, by the time I was able to order her a wheel chair she was only able to use it twice. The disease was progressing faster than I could find solutions, but I still felt proud that I did my best for her.

Christie talks about her pride in caring for her husband

Yes, I am proud of how I handled things. I shudder to think what would have been if I had not had the various strengths and skills I brought to the table. I needed to keep my own life going, and am thrilled that I was able to find creative ways to indulge my interests. It meant a lot of work for me but I'm glad I realized early on how important it was to make that effort. I'm proud of the fact that I knew myself so well and understood what would keep me nourished for this lengthy challenge.

In terms of the situations that helped me, I'm also thankful for the help I received from friends, Professional Caregivers, and other Family Caregivers who understood what I needed and were there to support me in the later stages of my husband's Alzheimer's.

Chapter 12

Hope for the present and possibilities for the future

Author's reflections:
The ability to have hope and bring to fruition the options that are available to us comes from our general view of the world. This is related to the matter of whether we are walking around seeing the glass half empty or half full. This ability goes beyond wanting something specific or having a particular expectation; both are given birth from a broader view of things. Seeing only the negative or feeling powerless about opportunities that are presented to us and therefore not taking any action towards what is being made available to us inhibits our ability to hope for the future or fulfill our dreams.

Hope in possibilities for positive outcomes is not based on wishful thinking or fanciful expectations that can never be met. It is more realistic.

When we fail to engage or be fully in the present, with our sights set only on the unfolding future, we may compromise our caring relationship, missing the experience of each and every moment.

And lastly, the hope for a better future cannot be based on a negative comparison to only the difficulties of the present, but more that the hope for better things to come is founded on the richness of this ability to live enthusiastically in the present with a full range of possibilities and experiences.

How do you think the future will compare to what you are experiencing now? Which aspects of the present fuel your hope for this future?

Suzanne talks about her hopes for the future in the context of her grief over the loss of her husband

Since my husband's death I've continued to be involved in a lot of organizations. That's what keeps me going. There are times that I have very low points and I don't think the future will get better. I call it depression, but I don't know if that's the right name. I miss my husband a great deal. For example, yesterday was both the day that my husband asked me to marry him and my half birthday. That's how I remember it. So yesterday was not a particularly good day for me.

Since I'm alone now, I try to have something to do every day to keep my spirits up. I don't really know what the future will bring. I am involved in the activities of the organizations I belong to, so that gives me something to look forward to, like conventions and travel. We are working on important projects like matching people who have lost limbs to top level prosthesis. This is very satisfying work for me. I get to see my friends whenever I go to work on these projects. That also gives me something to look forward to. I suppose I do generally think that things will get better for me.

Liz talks about the present and the future with her mother

The present is really good with my mom. We talk about everything and get together for special events and holidays and my whole family enjoys her company. She has a rich exciting life with classes and senior trips and I enjoy hearing about all of it. She is also active in her condominium complex and stays busy with all of the personalities and goings on there. I tell her all about my job and my kids and it really is a balanced relationship between us.

As my mother becomes more frail I'm guessing that the future will be much more complex than it is right now. Because I live the closest to her out of the four sisters, I'll probably be in charge when she needs more help. It will be difficult emotionally but I want to handle it with as much dignity and respect for her as I can. I think of our relationship as mutual care partnering rather than Caregiving, which to me has a more lopsided feel to it as a label.

I intend to continue to use humor and will encourage her to tell me everything so there are no secrets. All this is so that our future will unfold in the best way I know how. This has been working so far because I don't jump on her with all of my opinions and judgments when she tells me what is going on with her. Like when she fell, she confided in me that that scared her. Instead of my getting upset we calmly discussed a suggestion to get a Medic Alert button, but I let her decide. We ended up getting phones all over the place, and even on the floor. Additionally she got new shoes and she's going to physical therapy for balance. Plus she just lost 20 pounds with Weight Watchers, and that helped with everything. I don't think I would have even come up with all of these solutions if we hadn't discussed all the options together. She thought of most of them.

For the future, she brought it up that she's concerned that she won't be able to drive. This will be hard for all of us, but we'll manage. I could alter my work schedule to drive her around and she could also take cabs and buses. The problem I find generally with seniors I talk to at church is that they aren't willing to spend the money for alternative transportation even when it's cheaper than owning a car. Americans in general are very attached to their wheels so I suppose it's understandable.

Another issue is negotiating with her to also spend money now on important things that need replacing for the future. Because she doesn't know how long she will live and whether her money will hold out, it makes it hard for her to spend it. I feel that ultimately it's her money and she can do whatever she wants with it. She is generally conservative with finances except that she does enjoy her trips.

We discussed assisted living facilities and where she might like to live some day in the future. That would make things easier for her and for me if she becomes less able to live on her own. She has friends in different residences. I'll have to keep on top of the situation because there aren't always vacancies when you want them. I can see her staying in her home with hired help for a very long time. That would be the best future for all of us if nothing changes and then she wouldn't have to move.

The best ultimate outcome for her future would be to eventually die quickly one day without suffering. For my sake I hope it is a more gradual process so I can get used to the loss and say goodbye over time. It's going to be really tough for me. That part of my future I'm not looking forward to.

Musings on Mayeroff:

When we gaze out the window, looking forward to the wonders of spring, knowing that it follows the glories of winter and comes each year, the richness of the moment provides a sense of what is possible in the future.

In our caring we experience something as natural as the hope for the future blossoming in another's spirit and self-worth as we care for them in the present. Engaging fully in the tasks at hand, while feeling confident and creative allows us to hope that the future will unfold full of growth, interest and challenge.[39]

Author's reflections:
Our thoughts of the future are not always rosy, especially when we find ourselves in a tough situation, which we all know Caregiving presents. It's easy to get discouraged and when we become discouraged, we may start to doubt ourselves and our capabilities; we may despair and feel hopeless about the future, abandoning thoughts of a future of wellbeing.

Finding the small blessings in a situation, feeling proud of the ability to eventually solve difficult problems and knowing deep down that what we are doing for the person we are caring for is profound and beneficial to them on many levels allows us to see something positive. Finding the positive will allow us to also more easily see opportunities that we may have missed in our overwhelmed state. Experiencing more options and feeling less negative and trapped in our present helps us to grow a hope and confidence in our future.

Are you able to have hope, see opportunities and possibilities for now and for the future?

Suzanne talks about seeing possibilities for herself

I can see possibilities for both the present and the future. Basically I take one day at a time and don't postpone my happiness for a later day.

Liz talks about possibilities for now and the future with her mother

My mother and I have a really fun time together now. I like the way my mom approaches her death, her disability with the Rheumatoid Arthritis and getting sick generally. Her openness allows for a broad range of possibilities in our relationship in the present and for the future.

We talk about finances and religion. It's all out there, art, dance, news, the old days and any number of topics. I look forward to many more visits and conversations with her in the future. Since everyone else in the family is scattered all over the country, she is my tribe. She is from New York and familiar to me. When I moved to California all of that was erased. I certainly hope that our relationship will continue long into the future, but I'm realistic too. She's 84 years old, and I sort of know she won't be here forever. I don't need things to be better in the future. Even if they stay the way they are now with my mom I'd be happy.

Author's reflections:
As we get deeper into our Caregiving many of us hope that our loved ones' health will improve and that their futures will be easier. Another type of focus can bring hope for improvements that our caring will bring about. As we get better at our tasks we see how the world of opportunities opens for us and our loved one. Finding resources, getting help and sharing experiences are all opportunities that allow us to discover hope for our future. Putting aside the goals for physical health there is also the idea that building dignity in the person we are caring for or sharing our love with them can now become central themes in our caring and these pursuits can fill us with hope for a satisfying future.

Since Caregiving is a partnership, can you have hope that that partnership will become stronger?

Suzanne talks about the partnership with her husband

I felt that during the last five months of my husband's life we were a close partnership and we both had hope for our future. I had many low points because he was in and out of the hospital and did go to a nursing home for rehabilitation. I would get briefly depressed but having my daughter with me helped. I never really sat down and cried. His optimism helped me to stay hopeful.

I think it mattered a great deal to my husband that I was there during those last five months. He never said anything but I knew he was appreciative. When you ask what did my caring accomplish, it would have been terrible for him if we hadn't been there. He never would have been able to come home and I don't know what kind of care he would have gotten. I'm very proud of what my daughter and I did for him.

My view went back to my wedding vows of "in sickness and in health". Forty years later I was asked to act on the first part of those vows. Generally speaking we had great times when he was healthy, and when he was sick we usually got through it.

I can't have hope for our partnership to actually become stronger in the

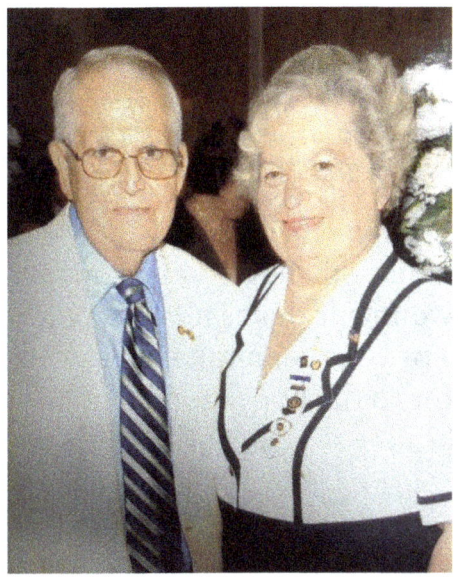

Suzanne and her husband

future because my husband passed away. What I can experience is a fuller understanding of the strong partnership we had. That understanding is what is becoming stronger. I feel stronger as a person knowing what I did to help my husband. As I travel through my life this strength gives me hope that I will have lots of new experiences and opportunities in the future.

Liz talks about her partnership with her mother

Yes, I have hope for both of us forming a stronger partnership in the future. I'm just glad she is open and honest. I do have to encourage her to share information. She comes from a world where you aren't supposed to worry anyone, especially your children. My goal for both of us is that in the future, we fully talk about things, put some perspective on things and keep the humor going. This is what I see as strengthening our partnership and ultimately that's what I am hoping for.

Musings on Mayeroff:

Believing that we would rise up to defend and protect those we are caring for fuels our ability to hope for their future. Without that belief we might be left to doubt that they would be able to make it through their struggles on their own.

Hope and courage go hand in hand. The more sure we are about our commitment to our caring, the easier it becomes to find the courage to overcome the difficulties we know we all will eventually face. Believing that we can courageously overcome difficulties and walk into a brighter future is what fuels our hope.[40]

Author's reflections:
Since the hope for the idea of having a future full of possibilities is built on the courage to actually move forward into those possibilities, we need to find that courage in the caring we are doing. Knowing that we will be there for the person we are caring for in times of difficulties adds to our ongoing sense of courage for facing the future and all of its possibilities.

When we commit to someone, whether it's early in a marriage, or, later on when that other person is in need, we often don't foresee how difficult things may become. Can you connect the depth of your commitment to the person you are caring for to the hope of making it through the tough times ahead?

Suzanne talks about experiencing tough times

I did make it through the tough times and came out to the life I have now. I know I had the commitment to my husband and promised my wedding vows to him, but truthfully I don't know if I would have the courage to go through all of that again. Although, God forbid, I would have to do it again, I'd probably do it. At least I hope I would.

Liz talks about tough times ahead with her mother

I know I have the commitment to care for her. I certainly have hope that we would make it through the tough times, just like we did with caring for my dad.
 What I really don't know is how much I'm going to miss her when she finally dies. That's a courage I'm not sure I'll have. I don't know how much loss I'll feel. I know I'll miss her but I don't know how much it will set me back. I don't have much hope that I'll get through the loss easily, that's for sure.

Liz talks about commitment to her husband

I feel the same way about my husband. It's hard to connect to the fact that there will be difficult times in the future. I didn't do much Caregiving for my husband when he had his prostate cancer surgery. My courage wasn't really tested. Now with the robotics he was up and around quickly. I did have to help with the long term side effects. I needed to have patience with his recovery in the areas of sexual and bodily functions. The only treatment was to have patience, keep trying. Having doctors who guided us helped. I suppose this help gives me some hope for the future that I won't be alone regardless of what happens.

Chapter 13
The challenge of the unknown

Musings on Mayeroff:
One of the most difficult things we find ourselves dealing with in life is facing the unknown. When we go into a caring relationship we are not leading but rather following another's lead. It's their disease, their crisis, their timeline, their treatment and their response to all that is happening to them that we are dealing with. In addition, Caregiving takes us away from the familiar and, often, we are faced with an unforeseeable future.[41]

Author's reflections:
Anyone who is attracted to control will tell you that they want to be sure that things will turn out the way they intend them to. It seems to make a lot of sense. In a world where you have control, actions lead to predictable results, and this feeling of certainty calms our anxious minds.

But life is hardly ever like that. Control is an illusion as is certainty. Truth be told, we are always living a life where anything can happen at any time, wresting our imagined control over a situation from us.

Eastern religions base many of their teachings on relinquishing control. We are asked to leave our attachments and desires behind. These wise teachers encourage us to live in the present moment so we can experience discovery and wonder and not try to orchestrate our future according to a rigid plan.

Caregiving, especially, is full of surprises. We are following another's path and adjusting to what they need from us. There is no certainty in this process; someone else is leading the way and we need to be flexible in following that lead. Trying to control the unknown, the road our loved one will be taking us down, leads to frustration and an unsatisfying Caregiving experience.

By following another's lead in our caring we leave behind some of our own comfort and head into unfamiliar territory. There is no way to know what lies ahead. How has facing the unknown helped you while caring for a loved one?

Patrice talks about not knowing how her autistic son would develop

My son and I have both grown through this process. I follow his lead because none of this was familiar to me before learning about his Autism and discovering who my son is. I had no preconceived ideas. I never realized I could work with someone the way I work with him and truly make a difference. I never realized I had this much patience. I never realized another person, even a child, could depend on you so completely. When we were first having him evaluated the speech therapist that came said in her report that we had our own way of communicating. She could observe that within the hour or so that she was here.

Years ago it was impossible to know how things would turn out with my son. Now that he has grown and acquired new skills he is able to communicate with everyone. His basic needs are always clear. So far he doesn't always do well with expressing his emotions. I don't know if he'll ever acquire these skills. In the meantime, my understanding him so deeply will continue to help him wade through the complications of communication and his emotions. I'm like his translator.

This summer started with a family cruise. I was not sure he would be able to handle any of it and this was certainly new territory for my whole family. Perhaps because he has grown more comfortable in new situations and acquired lots of new skills it turned out that he was fabulous, just a few small bumps along the way.

Marian talks about uncertainty in facing new situations with her husband

In the past my husband was the decision maker for how we would live our lives together. I enjoyed the decisions he made and had no trouble with that.

Because of his dementia I later became the decision maker. This was different for me. Even though I didn't know much about what I was facing I didn't run away and hide. I tried to imagine what he would have done in various situations we now found ourselves in. I tried to figure out what this or that decision would mean for our future. All of this was neither comfortable nor familiar to me but I faced it all willingly.

While I was a Caregiver there was a lot of uncertainty and I was unsure whether I was doing the right thing for him. There was no way to measure if I was right or wrong. It made me feel anxious and unsettled. On the other hand I was taking control of what I could and getting things done so I had two different emotions going on at the same time.

One of the things I followed his lead on even after his dementia started was on our religious participation like attending weekly mass. This didn't always work out for us because my health wasn't that great. Early on there was one time when I was sick and couldn't take him to mass. In his state of confusion he wrote an angry note that I suppose he was going to give to someone in charge about how I wasn't caring for him properly. He was threatening to drive himself to church but I had already taken away the keys to the car. From week to week I didn't know whether I would always be able to take him to mass but for the sake of his dignity staying intact I courageously tried.

Musings on Mayeroff:
When living with challenge both of us will change. Courage is an important factor in being able to meet the unknown.[42]

Author's reflections:
As we go through the complex world of Caregiving both the person we are caring for and we Caregivers will change. Sometimes we become more rigidly set into who we are and sometimes an entirely new side of our self appears. This can happen to either person.
  We all handle stress and an unknown future differently. We all handle uncertainty in our own unique way. Some of us will plunge into the unfamiliar situation with a fearless resolve and others of us will get all tangled up in fear, self doubt and anxiety.

Did the courage you had in facing the unknown lead to personal growth in your caring situation?

Patrice talks about growth in her son and in herself

Since we don't yet know the extent of what my son will ultimately be capable of we have bravely plunged in and are helping him acquire skills in any way we can. I never shy away from trying to introduce new concepts and skills to my son and I think that I have grown into a much stronger person as a result.
  My son is learning to speak and communicate, to share his emotions, though he doesn't always get it right just yet. I have been working with him on all this even though it's impossible to say when or if he'll understand a particular concept. This summer he has been phobic about weather and storms. Almost like the storms outside, I brace myself, batten down the hatches so to speak when my son is having an inner emotional storm. I deal with it, talk to him and then wait for a rainbow moment. When he can relax and enjoy something all the Caregiving culminates into something really beautiful. I know there will be another storm, but those moments are so worth it. Deep down I know if I backed off or lived in my fear for his future there would be many less of these rainbow moments.

Marian talks about her growth after her Caregiving ended

I had wanted to care for my husband as he struggled with dementia especially because I felt that he had had a terrible beginning due to growing up in the orphanage until he was seventeen years old. I didn't know in the earlier stages how hard it would become for me both on the physical and emotional levels. Because I wanted him to experience something loving no matter what was ahead of us I hung in there and did my best.
  The satisfaction of what I had given him was the main reason why I didn't cry when he died. Instead of sadness and loss I felt a deep satisfaction. It bothered me that I couldn't cry but I just didn't feel sad about the experience

of caring for him. I gradually started to bring this confidence into my life as a single woman and this eventually grew into a new feeling about myself.

Most of the rest of my own growth happened after I lost my husband. After he died I took a course that talked about how we become wiser as we age and that helped me to grow. Since I didn't have any idea of what lay ahead for me after being married for so many years, I found that I was enjoying the other people in the class and especially the teacher. I would consider that this course and some other new things I started to do supported my growth into a more confident person.

While I was my husband's Caregiver I was sort of on a plateau. We were never sure of where things were headed until the very end and I was just hanging on for dear life to get through each day. Once he was gone I finally could slowly start to realize and understand what I had accomplished. It was a proud feeling. I grew into a new idea of myself as strong and competent.

Musings on Mayeroff:
We base our ability to be courageous on our past experiences of facing the unknown, combined with being attentive to the present and doing what is needed.[43]

Author's reflection:
Depending on what we have experienced in our lives and how we have reacted to these experiences, we learn to be fearful or courageous. I remember hearing about two girls who were sharing their initial experiences with garden snakes. The first young girl saw a snake in the yard and ran screaming to the house. The second young girl saw her first snake and went over to it, watched it, eventually picked it up and brought it to her brother to show him. The first girl talked about how she had a lifelong fear of snakes while the second girl kept snakes as pets and never feared them.

We are always looking around to see whether the present situation feels safe. When we live a fear filled life we retreat and become more and more anxious. This vigilance most likely happens automatically on an instinctive level. Our imaginations run wild with frightening scenes of what could be.

In contrast when things have worked out well in the past we are fortified with courage for the future. When acting courageously was successful in the past it gets reinforced and we're willing to try it again in the new situations.

Have you ever been afraid because you didn't know what the future would bring? Describe a situation where this feeling came up.

Patrice talks about her fears concerning her son's future

I am always afraid I don't know what is around the bend. My son is growing and changing, but as a parent my ultimate goal is helping him to become independent. I still can't see that far ahead and be sure it is possible. That worries me almost constantly.

At times, like during his emotional upsets, I truly find myself worrying about the future. How can he go from these troubled times to independence? If he can't what will I do? What happens if something happens to me?

That can be a great deal of pressure. Then I take a step back and remember we have been here before. I remind myself that this is a phase that comes and goes. We will find a way through this challenge and there will be others and we'll get through those as well, somehow.

Marian talks about fear as she was suddenly given responsibility for the care of her father

I remember the time I was picking up my father in New York. He had dementia and my mother was his primary Caregiver. I would take him for the day each Saturday because it was my mother's busiest teaching day at the music school. It was important for me to help out so she could still earn some money.

This one Saturday she came up to the car and said "You have to take him. He's yours!" I asked her what she was saying. Did she want him to not live with her anymore? She said, "He scares me now." She had locked the doors of their apartment from the inside and he still tried to get out. This frightened her because she didn't know how to handle it. I asked her if I made any decisions would she support me? She said, "Whatever you want to do, you just do it."

I must say I was petrified. That whole day my husband and I didn't know what we were going to do about the situation. I struggled through calling people for help. At the time I had a lot of contacts with psychiatrists because of my work. We even called the police to see what could be done. They said that he would have needed to have committed a violent crime before they could intervene. In that circumstance they could take him to a mental hospital for observation.

Earlier in the day he had gone into the coat closet and taken out all of my daughters' hats and stacked them on his head to show us that he wanted to leave. We laughed when he came into the kitchen, and he laughed too, but the bottom line was that we knew he wanted to leave. We couldn't force him to stay with us and with four small children and a job; I wouldn't have been able to care for him anyway.

Once the police mentioned a mental hospital I realized I did have a contact who said she could get him into the state mental hospital nearby for observation. From there she would be able to get him into some sort of facility. We were able to take him over to the hospital that first day.

When we took him to the hospital they put him in a padded cell. I tell you that living through making that decision to leave him there was the most difficult thing I have ever had to do. My fear turned into regret. Luckily they were able to find him a room in the hospital section pretty quickly. He did realize that the other patients were mentally ill. I could tell by how he tried to describe them.

My mother had always been a force of nature to me and I generally feared her wrath. During all this I had no idea where all this would end or whether she would even accept what we had done. It turned out that in the end she actually was very grateful. For her it had been a traumatic experience to take care of him, especially by that point in his progression into pretty serious dementia. I started to see her less as someone to fear and more someone to feel sorry for.

Section C

What is there to learn in caring?

Chapter 14

Selflessness, loss of self and selfishness

Author's reflections:
Family Caregiving is built on the foundation of a lifelong relationship. Sometimes these relationships are healthy, warm and nurturing and sometimes they aren't. Parents can be selfless in the best sense as they create a life conducive to growth and filled with opportunity for their children. Some parents lose themselves in the relationship and end up depleted and drained as they struggle to meet all of their children's seemingly endless desires as opposed to needs. Others pay little attention to the emotional needs of their family as they pursue a more self-centered path of fulfilling their own desires. This happens frequently nowadays when someone becomes overly involved in their work, neglecting their relationships with families or friends.

Some relationships have clear boundaries between the parties and others are more invasive. The latter may be based on control or possession. Some relationships consist of separate, independent, fully mature humans and others are more parasitic where one incomplete person feeds off the other.

Musings on Mayeroff:
Sometimes conflict arises between taking care of ourselves and caring for another.[44]

Author's reflections:
There are often times when the Caregiver's choice boils down to, "It's me or them." When the interests of the Caregiver and the care receiver conflict there are no pat solutions. Something or someone has to give and it is usually the Caregiver who will need to make the bigger effort in resolving the conflict. This may mean sacrificing part of their own recognized needs and becoming more selfless.

Or, it might mean choosing to do something for themselves, although that may involve feeling guilty, selfish or feeling that they are not living up to the high expectations they have set for themselves as Caregivers.

Maintaining a balance between being selfish and selfless is a difficult issue for any Caregiver, especially when a loved one needs constant care. Have you been able to maintain this balance during your Caregiving journey?

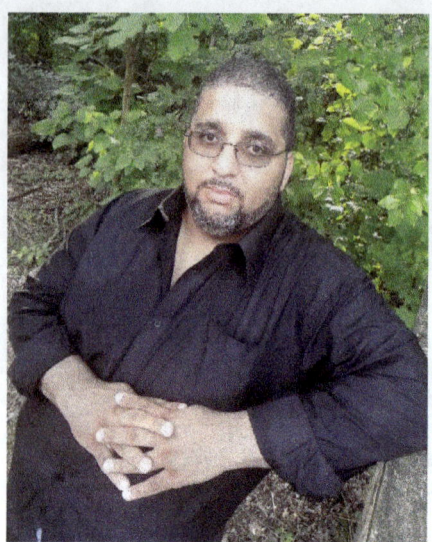

Chris F

Chris F. talks about keeping balance in his life while caring for his father

The only way I was able to keep any balance in my life and not feel selfish during the time we were caring for my father was to lose myself in my job. I felt I wasn't being selfish because I was caring for others at work. I was a new transit employee and at the same time I was a union representative. Rather than my getting lost in my caring for my father, it was a good outlet for me. Even though I could still help my father physically I ultimately couldn't change what was happening to him due to his Alzheimer's disease. He was getting worse in degrees and I realized I was losing him on several levels.

By becoming a union representative I could, at the same time as I was keeping my sanity more selflessly pay respect to my father. As a minister he was in the business of saving souls and now in my position, working for the union, I could save peoples' jobs. My concern was for the union members I represented. In a way I was saving the underpinnings of my fellow employees' lives, and I found myself identifying with who my father had selflessly been more and more. In reality that version of my father was no longer there. I felt that I was keeping it alive in my work.

As a union representative I felt effective, but with my father I was feeling more and more helpless. In a way it was also more selfish to give so much to my work even though I was helping people there. More and more I had to watch my mother struggle to take care of my father at home, and by then I had decided not to say anything to upset her. I felt that my voice was being lost at home but I could still speak out at my job to help others. It was a real conflict in me to handle what was going on.

Another way I kept balance in my life and didn't lose myself in my Caregiving was my study of martial arts. I didn't feel that this was selfish on my part. It was making me a better person to be involved in the arts. It changed my whole life. I had started with my teacher the year before my father was diagnosed and stayed with him for several years. My teacher had an almost physical resemblance to my father. He was a powerful and quite eloquent man just like my father. He became a father figure to me because the father I still had was no longer the same. I took private lessons and travelled with my teacher. I took seminars with him. For a while we were really close.

My job and my martial arts became my only comforts. Both diversions from my Caregiving ultimately taught me how to be a better Caregiver. I can see that now.

Sarah talks about keeping her life going as she cared for her mother

I was able to stay separate from her while I took care of my mother. I didn't lose myself in her care. I didn't feel selfish as I kept working. I also kept my relationship, and I was able to raise a child. I couldn't afford to get lost in caring for my mother because I had other responsibilities.

I was able to occasionally see friends but there was some disappointment there that they weren't taking good care of me. I needed more support from them and wasn't able to figure out how to get it. I don't think that needing more from them was being selfish either. I felt that I deserved help and support and my friends were either too busy or too self-absorbed to give it to me.

Sarah talks about members of her support group and their feeling selfish or lost in their Caregiving

Most of the people in my groups are able to continue to work as they care for their partners with cancer. They often become the bread winners…. In terms of feeling selfish they do struggle with the idea of whether it is OK to have friends, outside activities, go to a movie. I noticed that it was more rare to give themselves permission for those extra things outside of work. It might be OK to meet a friend for dinner but not OK to do something frivolous or escapist.

If the loved one needs constant care then the issue of getting a person in to take their place comes into the mix. Instead of feeling directly that they might be selfish to want a break, they would focus on whether this new person would be good enough at the caring. What they might be wondering deep down was did they really deserve a break? Could they leave and let someone else take over? Guilt was a part of it. Finding balance in their own lives became less of a focus. They were more reacting to the situation and often found themselves lost in their responsibilities and commitments.

Musings on Mayeroff:
When we are completely absorbed in something there is a loss of the separateness of ourselves from our activity. We merge with our singular purpose. We don't lose ourselves but rather can experience our deepest sense of who we truly are in the context of this work.[45]

Author's reflections:
Caring for another person brings about a very special partnership like a pas de deux in dance in which each partner plays a different role. Ideally the person being cared for takes the lead, creating the choreography and indicating how they want to be followed. The follower—or the Caregiver—then follows that lead, responding with split second precision. Beginners in both worlds often can't find that precision. They lose the beat, can't remember the steps or can't yet really share the dance as part of a partnership and may feel "lost" and out of sync.

On the other hand, getting "lost in the dance" is an entirely different experience. The dancers merge with each other and into the music, the space, the rhythm of their movements and time seems to disappear. This feeling usually takes years of practice to achieve.

Caregiving can parallel either experience. A Caregiver can feel lost and adrift, like a perpetual novice, or totally engaged and surrendered to their commitment to the other. There is no place for selfishness in this dance of caring when totally engaged and there is no place for loss of self either. This level of merging between two people transcends all that.

Are you able to feel totally engaged by your role as Caregiver, or do you sometimes feel lost and out of synch in it?

Chris F. talks about feeling mostly "lost" in the caring for his sister

I feel a little bit of both with my sister: once in a while I feel engaged with her care but mostly I am lost. My sister has been living with me for the last several years. She suffers with arthritis, a heart condition and she's also bipolar. Recently her arthritis has gotten worse and now she is asking to have a refrigerator and a microwave in her room. She is such a homebody already that this to me is a form of giving up. She never goes out, she doesn't come downstairs to cook anything and she sometimes even misses doctors' appointments. She thinks she knows more than the doctors because she looks things up on the internet.

I have to watch what I say; because of her being bipolar I could set her off and I don't want to deal with her anger. I had to watch myself with my mother but I never worried that my mother had a violent streak or would hurt herself. My sister is much more explosive and sometimes things would just come out of the blue. With my mother I could see things coming.

My sister goes from being incredibly exuberant to being incredibly sullen. There is no real in-between. There is about a half a second of transition and then she's in the opposite phase. For me I have to quickly switch gears between the extremes of her emotions. That's when I feel lost in caring for her. Earlier I hated being home but I realized that if I didn't get home she might really screw things up. There are times when I'm so exhausted from the situation that I get home and basically pass out.

She came to live with me about six years ago to help take care of our mother. All was well and good at first because I had no clue about the issues I now know about. As things began to surface I wondered what I had gotten myself into. I had taken care of my father and then my mother and now it looked like I would have to take care of my sister. I definitely didn't volunteer for this. I feel like it was thrust onto me.

To this day she hasn't acknowledged any understanding of how hard it has been for me to be around her. I'd leave for work in the morning and come back to find she had overturned all the furniture in the living room. When I would ask her about it she felt it was her right because she was angry and that's how she needed to express it.

Sarah talks about feeling engaged as she cared for her mom

I did feel committed and engaged when I took care of my mother. I felt good about it and felt that I had done what could be done for her. I was proud of the fact that I could be nice to someone who hadn't been very nice to me. The fact that I just did it and didn't question or second guess myself makes me proud as well. I was in sync with her needs and it felt right to be doing this for her. There was no one else who could or would step up to do what I did for her.

Musings on Mayeroff:
When we care for another we have a heightened awareness of their needs, we observe our responsiveness and how we use our personal resources. We are needed by another, so they can make it through the day or flourish; our caring for them becomes an expression of our inner selves.[46]

Author's reflections:
Watching Caregivers do their job is like watching parents minding children on the playground. There is a constant monitoring and then responding to rapidly arising situations. In an ideal situation the Caregiver gets to use all the things they are naturally good at to assist them in their caring. They watch their loved one benefit from this care. They too benefit by experiencing satisfaction from this caring relationship.

How does it feel to be needed and to respond selflessly?

Chris F. talks about being needed by the employees in his union

I was once told that I had a Caregiver's makeup and I should become an Emergency Medical Technician. It feels good to do my job as a Union Representative. Sometimes it was even an ego boost when things went well. I had to be careful not to let it become an ego trip because then it would no longer be a selfless act on my part. I believe that when much is given, much is required. The margin for error is clear. If I am weak in a negotiation then others will suffer. If I can't be strong for others then they will be trampled upon by others who are stronger than them--like our bosses. I need to bring all my strengths and talents to bear in each situation.

Sometimes it feels good to be needed but sometimes it feels like the whole world is on my shoulders and my feet are in quicksand. Sometimes it can be a rewarding job and sometimes it can be a thankless job. Either way I can't afford to be having an off day because others will lose liberties and suffer as a result. I feel pressure from the other union members because they don't want to lose and I feel pressure from management because any weakness on my part is like blood in a shark pool for them. I am always tap dancing as a negotiator in the defense of workers' rights even when I feel that they may be controversial. I must selflessly put my own judgments aside and do what I can for my union members.

In being needed I feel the call of duty but I also feel the fear of failure. There will also be a day when I'm no longer working in the union office and I realize that others will remember me, good, bad or otherwise.

Sarah talks about weighing her selflessness against her own needs

At the basest level it feels good to be needed. There's almost a feeling of being superior to the person who needs you because you can fulfill their needs when you selflessly put your own needs aside. I feel that this is a better position to be in. It's what I do for a living so it is very familiar. I chose my profession because caring is what I did as a child.

I don't, however, like to be the Caregiver for my friends. It's hard to be this way all the time with everyone. I can't be selfless all the time. I need to have equal relationships with my friends of give and take.

Musings on Mayeroff:
We care for another for their own sake and not merely as a means to become ourselves.[47]

Author's reflections:
What draws most Caregivers to their role is certainly not what they are going to get out of it. Most take on the role in a selfless way, at least at first. They are concerned primarily with the wellbeing of their loved one. Any benefits they derive come about organically as the side effect of the work they do and through the caring they are able to show.

Do you experience your role as a Caregiver as a time to also take care of your own needs, or is it a time to limit your focus to your Caregiving?

Chris F. talks about dating at the same time he was grieving for his dad

When I was caring for my dad, I dated but I could not direct myself towards a proper relationship or focusing on those needs. But at least I was able to go out for some companionship. After my father passed I was in such a state of mourning that I became totally lost in my job as a union representative. I still couldn't focus on my needs. I had been seeing someone and we liked each other, but to escape the feelings of losing my dad, my job came first. She finally reminded me that my job wouldn't keep me warm at night and I let her slip through my fingers. There were other relationships that I could have had, but the fact that I was in mourning for my dad didn't let me see the possibilities until it was too late. By then I had lost so much.

About three years later I finally came to the realization that I had to start living for myself again. I understood that I had been chasing a ghost and in terms of my job I had set it up that I couldn't afford to fail. That was part of why I felt that I couldn't become distracted by a relationship. The job had become my mistress, and the way that I was fulfilling the memory of my father. His job as pastor of a church and my job as union representative had many similarities in the ways that we both helped people in their time of need. Once I realized that I needed to get on with my own life I started taking my dating more seriously.

Sarah talks about keeping her own identity as she cared for her mother

I think that it is harder to lose yourself when caring for a parent, and I didn't when I cared for my mother. It seems more likely to get lost if it is your spouse or partner. As I cared for my mother I also kept a focus on my own needs. For example I kept a routine with my mother and instead of always going over to her place I would call so I could continue to have a life at home with my family.

Chapter 15

Having goals while living in the moment

Musings on Mayeroff:
When we are grounded in the present moment we can truly tend to another's needs. The final outcome of caring therefore takes a back seat to the process of that caring in the moment.[48]

Author's reflections:
Sometimes we become too goal oriented, living our days always looking towards achieving a future goal. We wish we were already there, a place of comfort after having attained our goals. This can make us restless in the present, prohibiting us from living fully in our life as it unfolds.

Most of us enjoy taking vacations, regarding them as pleasant breaks from the day-to-day routine. The problem comes when our only pleasure derives from vacations or weekends and we see the rest of our time as a "daily grind."

The same can be said for a large purchase. Sometimes we wear ourselves down to be able to afford a big house or fancy car and no one asks if achieving the goal was worth all the sacrifice. We all have dreams for our future, and that's positive, but if we forget to be present, living "the now" to the fullest, finally attaining that future goal may just lose its import and source of gratification for all we lost along the way.

How are you at organizing and taking care of your day-to-day affairs? Do you enjoy it as a process?

Alicia talks about enjoying the process of preparing for her private yoga students

I enjoy the entire process of teaching Yoga and caring for my students. I take pleasure right from the initial contact with a new student to their final class with me. In terms of my overall goals I don't see it that I'll have my private Yoga clients forever. Generally speaking I see that I'll have them for a period of time, they'll be empowered to know what they have to do for themselves and then they will leave the nest. However in my teaching I focus entirely on what is needed during each step of their journey and not on this final outcome.

Before they come in I prepare the physical space, clean it, and organize it. I might add a candle and music to create the right environment. In terms of

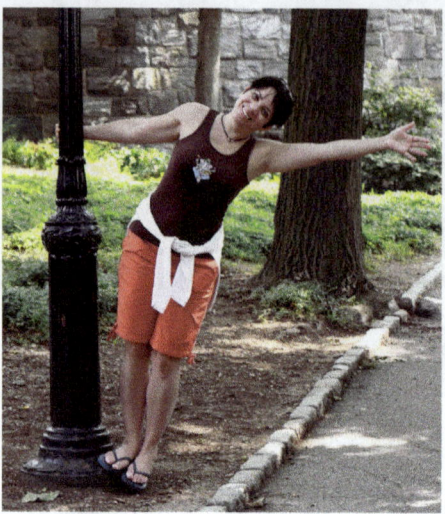

Alicia

my own process I take about 15 minutes to calm and center myself before we start so I don't hit them with my daily craziness. In addition I've already researched their condition long before they arrive on my doorstep.

I always start by asking the person how they are feeling right now and this may alter my approach for that day. An example might be if the person is really in a lot of pain I want to do something with them that will lessen the pain and help them feel better right away. If they are doing well then I'll stick to the lesson plan for that day. Yoga by its very nature puts an emphasis on the process and doing the movements with focus and attention. I don't push my students by setting up goals beyond doing each posture as best as they can for that day in that moment.

Terry talks about enjoying the process of caring for her dad

I really enjoy the process part of my work and I'm good at it. I'm a project manager at my job and that's what I love to do.

With my dad I dove deeply into the day to day process of his care. With his care the bulk of these daily processes for me came down to journal, journal, journal.....from the first moment my Dad was diagnosed I started a Microsoft document to record everything. I put dates, names and contacts, discussions, results of tests, what was the next step. Day by day, every appointment was recorded. I put everything on paper. One page had all the drugs he was on. Another page had all the dates of all the tests he had, where he had them and what doctor prescribed it. The rest was a journal of what doctors he had been to, what procedures they performed and what they said. It turned into a book.

On the financial front I started the process of helping my dad hand over his financial information to my mom to make her life a bit easier after he was gone. I told my dad that it was for my mom, and I got him to write down all the financial institutions where he had accounts. Who should she contact, what were the account numbers? I also thought to present it to him as keeping the assets that he worked so hard for. I was able to phrase it in such a way that he could feel honored and respected and we could gather the information we needed.

During this entire time there was very little focus on my part on what was ultimately happening to my dad with his terminal cancer. I suppose I used my focus on the day to day processes as a way to cope with knowing deep down that I was ultimately losing my father.

Author's reflections:
When we are on the path towards our goals there is the path itself, and then there is the direction in which the path is leading us towards its end. Some paths are direct while others are more roundabout. Reminding ourselves of what the goal is can get us through tough situations and motivate us to keep going along our path no matter the route.

Athletes set goals; whether it's that finish line to cross or a personal challenge to be met, they are motivated by these goals. When the present—their training, diet and other extraneous matters, etc.—is arduous, keeping their "eyes on the prize" will help see them through.

Similarly, starting a new business can seem daunting at first; there may be some rough going in the process, but keeping the goals for the business in mind can be essential to the success of the start-up.

In Caregiving, our goal may be to keep the person we are caring for emotionally stable as their physical state starts to deteriorate. Finding ways to entertain or enrich them and keep their mind occupied during this process is a way to achieve this goal.

As a caring person and/or a Caregiver are you goal oriented?

Alicia talks about being a privately goal oriented person

In my own life I have blinders on about achieving my goals but I am not one to talk about them or brain storm with others. My husband likes to talk about the different aspects of his plans but I don't. I have those conversations with myself inside my own head.

So when I say I have a 5 year plan it means I already have a 5 year plan. It's something I made up in my head and it is something that is going to happen. I take the time to think about how I am going to make this happen. How will I pull together the resources to make it happen?

The reason I don't brain storm with others is that I feel that I am imposing my uncertainties on them. The only one I feel comfortable brain storming with is my mentor. She is different from others in that she is open and non-judgmental and has very good boundaries to let me know when she has time for me. With her I don't feel that I am imposing. She also tells me when there is something she cannot help me with, and that I'll have to work this out myself.

Alicia talks about being goal oriented while caring for her private yoga students

During my work with my students I am totally immersed in the process but I also hold an overall goal for them in my mind. I have a place that I want them to reach but at the same time I know it is completely up to them.

I know I can be the best teacher in the world with the best tools in the world but if the person doesn't apply those tools it won't work. I can't be with my students 24/7 to check on them. I also have to be careful with my language not to communicate that it is their fault for their not getting better. I support their choices no matter what. I love to see their eyes light up when I make a minor adjustment in their posture, like how they are holding their head. Suddenly after all the pills and different things that they have tried they are finally pain free. That experience drives me forward, being able to help to give that to someone.

I have a teacher that lives according to the philosophy that yoga isn't about touching your toes. It's what you learn on the way down. I have found that that philosophy can take many forms.

Terry talks about being goal oriented while caring for her father

I am very goal oriented. For the big picture I was determined that my dad should get the best care possible and choose the best treatments. I wanted to make sure we were making knowledgeable choices and talking to the right people. It was a matter of doing the research, asking the right questions and always getting more information.

Terry talks about caring for her mother as the entire family cared for her father

I also had the goal that my mother wouldn't be left out in the cold regarding our father's care and would have our full support since she was the primary Caregiver. I also wanted to make sure she would have a break. She was in their apartment together with him 24/7. She found it difficult to leave him, even to go to the grocery store or the bathroom because her fear was that he would die or something would happen while she was gone. My goal was to give her some time away from the situation.

In order to support our mom we would also monitor my dad's being abusive and tell him to stop. An example was that he didn't want her to cook because he didn't like the smells. She would be crying when we arrived because she knew he needed to eat and didn't know what to do for him. We would talk to him and sympathize with his struggles but remind him that we are people too and he needed to work with us to provide his care. The only one my father would really open up to was my brother so when he needed a talking to we'd instruct my brother in what was happening. Then he would share what was on all our minds with my dad.

Author's reflections:
The trajectory of our lives is entwined in the past, present and future, the present being the central glue that holds everything together. When we think of our past history and future hopes we are able to see more possibilities for the present. What we are doing now gives meaning to where we came from and where we are headed. It's our story and ultimately all parts are needed to make it complete. The present allows us to give meaning to the past and creates insights that we may have missed at the time we lived it. The present also allows us to have more choices for the future based on who we are, how we are living and what our goals are.

How are you at staying "in the moment"?

Alicia talks about staying in the moment while she was taking care of her mother

Taking care of my mother was a mixture of duty and knowing that she was dying. We knew she had cancer, and that by the time I was caring for her there was nothing we could do about curing it. I wanted to share her experience and have time with her. It wasn't that I was trying to fix my relationship with her, but more that I didn't want to have any regrets in the future. I knew that the only way I would feel comfortable was to stop my life and move down with her for the last three months of her life. I felt that I did what I needed to do and I feel good about it.

I realized that I could be with her and put aside our past relationship and in addition that I wasn't overly concerned with her death. So in answering the question, yes I could experience being in the moment with her. The history of our relationship wasn't great but during those last three months all that didn't feel important anymore. This was the person who gave me life and now she was dying. I felt compelled to be with her. I didn't feel like I could guide her in her dying process because even though I read a lot of books about it, I still didn't really understand the process. I more felt that I needed to witness her experience.

I also needed to be there because my father wasn't in touch with the reality of the situation and he kept pushing her to have more treatments against all the doctors' recommendations. In contrast to how I was approaching the situation, he could not be in the moment with what was happening with my mom probably due to his fears. I felt that I needed to protect my mother against all the external harm he wanted to bring to her body. What I felt she really needed was to prepare for the process of leaving her body. Helping her with this process kept me focused on the experience as it unfolded so I could really share it with her as much as was possible.

Terry talks about being in the moment with her dad

I can be tenacious and stay in the moment if I have to figure out something or solve a problem. Examples would be … finding a doctor, getting approval for a test or getting the insurance to pay for something. I was right there figuring it out.

I never allowed myself to worry about the future and think, Oh my God, he has lung cancer and is dying. I can reflect on my experience as his Caregiver but I still don't think I have grieved yet for his loss and let go of the emotion that is still inside me. I stay in the moment now by gradually letting the grieving process happen over time. One way I can work on this is with the slides we have of my dad when he was alive. I've been making them digital and can make books for my relatives with all of his photos. It's helping to process the loss and keeps me in the moment by giving me something to do for my family to be able to share in his memory.

Chapter 16

Can I care and can the other be cared for?

Musings on Mayeroff:
Not everyone is capable of caring for another. Caring is a special gift requiring certain skills and forbearance that not everyone has.[49]

Author's reflections:
It is not enough to want to care for someone else or to wish for the other person's growth and fulfillment. The Caregiver must also know and practice those behaviors and interventions that make Caregiving of benefit to both themselves and the person they are caring for. It's important to remember that Caregiving entails, not only the physical, visible, day-to-day act of "giving care," but an emotionally charged relationship with unforeseen obstacles. Often, the Caregiver will be the one having to work harder and with more awareness focused towards overcoming difficulties.

Do you feel that you have the skills required to be a Caregiver? What skills do you have that allow you to be a successful Caregiver?

Susan talks about her skills as a Caregiver and with her husband

I do feel that I have the skills required to be a good Caregiver. I have done a lot of research into the disease of Alzheimer's, so I have in mind what might need to be done as my husband reaches each new stage of illness. I think I am doing well because I can see how my husband responds. If I need to change, I do.

My overall curiosity and positive outlook concerning what is happening are also skills I bring to the situation. I have always had an interest in people with special needs. Setting aside the overall tragedy of my husband's illness, I find the journey fascinating. For example it was interesting to me to see how he reacts to different medical situations and how his brain operates so differently from mine as he copes with everything.

Barbara talks about her Caregiving skills in her work and with her husband

I know that I was a good Caregiver for my husband during his cancer and

I now use my skills in my profession to help other Caregivers. I'm a good listener. I reflect on what is needed and I'm analytical so I can divide tasks into manageable jobs. I'm also result oriented.

I only worry about specific things. Ironically, even after losing my husband from cancer, I don't worry about my health. In the past I worried about my husband for many years and intuitively had a feeling before it happened that he would get sick. I do have to let myself off the hook about self-fulfilling prophesy and his illness. I can't worry like that anymore. I limit my worries to things I can manage or change. It's an important skill that I communicate to my clients.

As I look back I can say that I was an intuitive Caregiver beyond anything logical. One time we had a screaming match about what my husband was eating. I accused him of trying to kill himself and he said out loud "Don't you think I would know it if I were going to die?" The fact was that he had probably already had the cancer at this point and would be dead a mere six months later. So I suppose my intuitive Caregiving was more refined than his take on the situation. My worries about him were based on this intuition.

Barbara talks about using her Caregiving skills with her clients

Everyday my clients say to me "I don't know how you thought of that, I didn't know where to start." I have a skill of keeping my clients in the moment and not projecting them too far ahead.

I'm working with a husband right now who thinks he is being the ultimate Caregiver. He loves his wife who has very significant health issues. As we spoke I realized that in spite of what kind of job he believed he was doing he had a real lack of information about what was happening. I could also see that he had no documents, healthcare proxy, do not resuscitate orders, etc. I also knew that his goal of being a competent Caregiver would be impossible to reach without understanding what these documents meant and then creating his own set. Because I'm analytical I had the overview and could break things down so he wasn't overwhelmed and could have a plan.

Author's reflections:
There are degrees of caring. Not everyone is in a position to grow and flourish emotionally or spiritually while they are being cared for. Some people recover from their diseases and injuries and others can't. No matter the extent of the challenges some take on the challenge with courage and others feel depressed and defeated.

Some care is more custodial, especially when physical needs are of primary concern. A Caregiver must remember that, no matter the condition or mood of the person being cared for, they deserve to be allowed to maintain their dignity and to be treated respectfully. A person under care is often capable of demonstrating their ability to flourish by their uplifted moods, even finding peace. This mostly occurs when in the hands of a skilled Caregiver who is deeply involved in their care. Some degree of love is almost always a factor and the depth of the caring often demonstrates the extent of that love.

Do you have an interest to comfort the person you are caring for even when their personal growth is not possible?

Barbara talks about how she cared for her Caregiver client even though his personal growth wasn't happening

Initially I questioned whether I would even take this one case. I had to adjust my expectations about what I think my job is. When this client hired me I was very clear with him that I can help to clarify what is going on, but I won't be able to change the outcome.

He is not able to comprehend the disappointment and the reality of his situation with his wife's failing health. All I can do is remind him of the truth of the physical situation with his wife. I draw a line in the sand for what can be hoped for with her.

He feels that I am on his team and his challenge is whether he will finally trust what I am telling him and grow into the realities that he is facing on his own. I can live with being a comfort for him whether he grows or not. I feel good that he knows he has me on his team.

What abilities do you have that set you apart from others and allow you to assume the care of another?

Barbara compares her organizational skills to the lack of that skill in her client.

There's the idea of organization when it comes to being a Caregiver. When I walked into my client's house he showed me a bunch of envelopes from different doctors. I told him that he would need a book to help keep everything organized. Right then, instead of waiting until he understood what the whole project would involve, he left the room to go off to look for a book. He wants to accommodate and oblige but he has no sense of organization. He's all over the place. He wants immediate answers to his questions but doesn't have the organizational skills to keep a good history.

In contrast, when I cared for my husband, I had a book for his records and everything was very organized. I could also hear the objective information the doctors were giving me and didn't distort things. I also knew which questions to ask and how to analyze the answers. These skills were all different from my client's. It's funny, but I'm realizing that I don't remember any of my husband's information now. I've forgotten all the names of the medications and the lab test numbers.

Susan talks about being a skilled Caregiver

I know that other people don't have the skills to be good Caregivers, but I feel that I'm very good at it. I have many coping abilities that others lack and that allow me to be a good Caregiver. Several examples of my skills are that I am generally a positive person and don't dwell on the negative; I am very flexible and can change things as needed; I am also very good at multi-tasking so I can quickly move from one task to another.

Musings on Mayeroff:
One of the most important aspects of caring, experienced but rarely spoken of, is the acceptance of that care by the other person.[50]

Author's reflections:
Is the person you are caring for receptive to your care? Do they consider your suggestions to improve their situation? Are they working towards the same goals for themselves that you are for them? These may become sticking points between Caregivers and their loved ones. Being on the same page, so to speak, about these issues is important for a strife-free relationship; if not, Caregiving may become fraught with unresolved antagonisms.

Does the person you are caring for let you take care of them or is there resistance?

Barbara talks about parenting her son

My son is the perfect mixture of the neediest person you've ever met and the most resistant person you've ever met. His neediness is based on the fact that he has his father's DNA and his resistance is based on the fact that he also has his father's DNA. He is presently experiencing age appropriate difficulties in trying to focus. For example when I ask him to do his homework he careens wildly from one topic to another. It's hard for him to settle down.

I need to help him in this area so that he gets done what he needs to do. He's a smart, competent, accomplished kid. Lately he's really lost his grasp. I want to care for him but he's resisting the care. I find myself totally losing it.

I try to provide him with the cues that he hasn't been able to figure out on his own. Verbally he says he understands and he wants to learn how to do better. By the next day it's like the conversation never happened, the confrontation never happened, the information was never given.

When he doesn't hold on to anything I tell him I feel totally impotent. My anger and frustration start to enter the picture and my communication becomes so charged that I wonder if I'm not shutting him down at the same time that I'm attempting to care for him and make things better. My delivery becomes aggressive and confrontational instead of loving and generous. No one is benefitting from the way things are now.

Susan talks about her husband

With my husband's Alzheimer's he generally lets me care for him and will even ask for assistance with a task such as dressing. I sometimes wait to intervene because I think he might resist, but then find he does accept my assistance more readily than I thought he might.

Chapter 17

The commitment of caring

Author's reflections:
It takes commitment to care for another. When we take on the responsibility of Caregiving we also take on the dedication and loyalty to the person we are caring for. It isn't necessary to move in with the person to become their Caregiver but there does need to be a commitment to the overall task.

Peter Whybrow's book American Mania opines that, as inheritors of various traits from our nomadic ancestors, travel is in our nature, even if it means separating families by large distances. In our busy, mobile, noisy, distracted world our ability to commit to someone who is frail or disabled, which studies show can take anywhere from 10 to 60 hours a week, in many ways becomes more difficult.

It starts with a society where you can hop on a plane as easily as going to your favorite restaurant, so families no longer feel the imperative to remain physically close; now, loved ones are only a plane ride, phone call, text message or email away but have we considered what would happen if illness strikes one of us? There is good reason to reflect on what our commitment to each other would be.

Initially our commitment to our parents and siblings is challenged when traditional holiday time comes and we are not "back home." Hugs don't travel well over phone lines or in emails. Distance apart also prevents the newer members of the family, such as the grandchildren, nieces and nephews, from even getting to know each other. It is a rare family where grandma and grandpa live in the apartment upstairs, mom and dad in the middle and the grandkids in the finished basement downstairs.

The problem of living far apart becomes even more acute when illness strikes either those who stay or those who have left. When those of us leave the family nest, we may find new neighborhoods, new friends, but no one to step in to help when things start getting tough. That was when family members would traditionally have cared for each other in the past. And, for those we've left behind, when help is needed it is a challenge for them to find the kind of care they would have previously expected from us or other close family members.

Our futures depend on our ability to create these committed, tight knit and supportive communities again. All over the country there are movements afoot to do just that. Livable Communities, Aging in Place and Time Sharing organizations are all working towards replacing a lifestyle of being committed to each other through our family networks that has mostly been lost.

These organizations are building communities where they organize specific ways for neighbors to start caring for each other again. Faith based groups, community and service organizations also have taken up the slack that our families used to fill. If it means organizing transportation for those who can no longer drive for trips to the local supermarket or pharmacy these community groups find committed members to offer these and other services to seniors or citizens who are disabled.

How have these times of hyper-mobility changed your life and your commitments to your family?

Claudine talks about her far-flung family

There is no one in our extended family that lives nearby. My immediate family, consisting of my husband and daughter, is isolated from the rest of our larger family. My daughter has her own apartment about a ½ hour away.

My cousins live in Canada, and my closest relationships are with my other cousins who live in France. I'm in touch with them through email on a regular basis. They stay in touch by sending me photos. I feel like I belong to this extended family but only through technology. I don't feel deeply committed to any of my cousins nor would I leave my family to care for any of them if they were seriously ill.

When my husband developed diabetes and my daughter was having her recent health issues the three of us became closer but it may have had something to do with knowing we are all we have. No one is going to watch my husband's blood sugar and make sure he eats well besides me. No one is going to take my daughter to her doctor for tests and keep up with her latest health news besides her parents. We seem to have circled the wagons around each other when it comes to our health issues and caring for each other.

Christie talks about her lack of a serious commitment in both her and her husband's family due to both busy schedules and living at a distance

My entire family moved to the west coast of the United States. They are spread out from California and Oregon to Alaska. I was the only person in my family who stayed behind to care for my Grandmother in New York when she was alive. I was very committed to her and cared for her before she died during the three years that she suffered with a broken hip and then colon cancer.

I was mostly on my own during the eight years I cared for my husband with his cancer and Early Onset Alzheimer's. Not one of my busy sisters or parents was able to even visit during those tense times. We spoke on the phone and I would take my husband for visits to see them on the west coast, but that was the extent of our commitment as a family. There was no real willingness on the part of my family to change or uproot their lives and families to help me in any substantial way.

My husband's older brother lives in New York City with his wife and both are busy professionals. They helped me take care of my husband when they could. In terms of the rest of his family my husband came from a small family and he and his brother didn't keep much contact with their cousins in Oklahoma. My brother-in-law has one daughter and two sons but we only saw them during the holidays. I was only able to call on his side of the family one afternoon a week when my husband started showing more intense signs of Alzheimer's so I could continue to go to work. It wasn't much time in the overall scheme of things but it helped.

My mom had the same issue with this lack of commitment from our family with my dad in California. He had dementia overlapping the last six years of my husband's Alzheimer's. There was only one daughter out of four who lived in town and could help my mother with my dad. Hospice stepped in during the last year or so. We would all visit but she had the brunt of his care. It wasn't easy for her especially because her health wasn't good. Rheumatoid arthritis had affected many of her joints and destroyed the strength in her hands.

My sisters have husbands, children and now grandchildren but I see them only rarely. There is very little commitment beyond each one's immediate family. One of my sisters in Oregon had breast cancer and her husband and son had to take care of her on their own during her treatments. Earlier she had been on her own when she cared for her husband who has Scleroderma, an autoimmune disease and after his heart surgery. In addition her brother-in-law and two step-sons are all dealing with drug addictions and she and her husband have been coping with the fall out over the years. None of the rest of our family has committed to be there for my sister beyond our phone calls.

Musings on Mayeroff:
Caring develops over time and needs to be consistent.[51]

Author's reflections:
One of the lovely things about the internet is that it connects long lost friends and relatives. You just have to search for a name and that friend, relative or old acquaintance magically reappears in your life. In years gone by you would have had to pay a detective to locate your missing cousins in Oklahoma or schoolmates with changed names and distant or exotic addresses.

After the initial flurry of exchanges about your new life and theirs, then what? Do you pick up where you left off all those many years ago, having bonded anew, or do you go back to a more impersonal arrangement, getting in touch every few years or so? According to Mayeroff, for true caring to happen with all of the many facets we have been discussing in this book there has to be a renewal of the commitment to each other and an active involvement in each other's lives.

There are many examples of stories where this renewal to the commitment of the original relationship occurs. High school sweethearts meet years later and become lovers. Best friends travel together and still enjoy their ability to finish each other's sentences and laugh at the same absurdities they enjoyed as children. And more and more as we grow older these relationships become the ones we can count on as we age and become frail. This is the reason we are starting to include Informal Caregiver as the nomenclature to describe these friends caring for friends. It is no longer only a family member who will step into this role of Caregiver. Sometimes it is a neighbor next door and other times it is a person from the past who might demonstrate this strong sense of commitment to a friend in need.

Do you know anyone who has become an Informal Caregiver? Do you know anyone who is deeply committed to someone they had lost contact with for a long period of time?

Christie talks about neighbors caring for neighbors

I've met a woman who is caring for her neighbor in their condominium. They are great friends and now that he is frail and has many health issues she has taken on the role of Primary Caregiver. He no longer speaks with his son and there are no other family members left to care for him. This woman has recruited other members of her condo to help with certain tasks and they are all deeply committed to the wellbeing of this friend. He has always been quite social and other old friends of his have offered to visit and take him to lunch. This Informal Caregiver arranges for transportation, oxygen and wheelchairs so that he can stay involved with these friends of his. She also makes sure he is fed and clothed along with taking care of some of his financial affairs. He is not paying her for any of this, nor does she expect him to.

Christie talks about re-united sweethearts during illness

I know of a sister of one of my friends who got married late in life to her high school sweetheart. They had lived across the country from each other for most of their adult lives and hadn't seen each other in years. Neither had married. Once they found each other again at their high school reunion they immediately rekindled their passion for each other and were married a few months later.

When she developed cancer after their blissful fifteen years of marriage he stood by her side as her Caregiver. He lovingly cared for her over several years until her death.

Chapter 18
Guilt and neglect

Author's reflections:
When we hear Caregivers describing their feelings of guilt the normal instinct that most of us have is to comfort them and remind them of how much good they are doing. It seems crazy to us that a Caregiver would feel guilty about asking the person they are caring for to make their own tea or wait until tomorrow for a haircut. We don't want to see Caregivers experiencing the uncomfortable feelings and emotional pain of guilt in addition to everything else they are going through.

Milton Mayeroff sees things differently. Just as pain is an alarm coming from our physical being, he believes that guilt is also an alarm in our emotional lives, a call to action and to our problem solving capabilities. The feeling of guilt invites us to say there is something not right here, and it needs fixing.

I had not thought about it like this before nor had I read it anywhere else. He challenges us to examine just how we do care for another, allowing ourselves to find those possible instances where we have neglected the person we are caring for; once the challenge is met and corrected, suggests Mayeroff, we will be able to renew our pledge of Caregiving in a more engaged manner, being more sensitive to the needs of another and looking for ways to meet them.

It is also important to note that when we feel guilty for something harmful we have done to the person under our care, we need to examine very closely why and how it was done, whether intentional or inadvertent, and perhaps seek out professional help to help us work through the problem so that it will never happen again. This renewed determination will help us to turn failings such as abuse, inattention or neglect around. A new outlook such as this helps, too, to allay those nagging feelings of guilt.

Musings on Mayeroff:
Guilt is an internal alarm that requires our attention. If I can feel it deeply enough, understand its origins and accept that we can all, do things we'll later feel guilty about, it gives us the opportunity to change things and strengthen our commitment to the other person.[52]

Author's reflections:
Rather than rationalize our guilt away we can look at its source for inspiration. It may mean changing something about ourselves or changing how we are treating the person we are caring for. This push to make things better gives us a chance to experience the fullness of our Caregiving because we are growing through the process.

Sometimes the feeling of guilt is a reminder to get back to our caring and renew our appreciation of our role. Has there been a time when you felt guilty or neglectful about something you had done or not done in your caring for another?

Liz talks about guilt waking her up to realize how complex the care for her mother-in-law would be

My mother-in-law came to live with us in the early stages of her dementia and during her long time addiction to pain killers. I thought I could handle her care because I was home and wasn't working at the time. It made sense on the surface of things.

In terms of guilt, after she was with us for a short while I had witnessed her fall into our couch in the living room. I didn't think much of it at first because it was soft and happened slowly. I didn't realize that there was something I might be neglecting to see. It turned out she had broken her rib. She didn't appear to be in any extra pain but then the pain killers she had been addicted to for many years might have been masking it. At first I felt some guilt but in the end I don't consider anything I did as being intentionally neglectful but rather that this entire situation was way beyond my abilities and I didn't realize it at first.

The guilt I was feeling in missing her medical condition was a wakeup call for me. That was the point when I realized that I'm not qualified to be her Caregiver or to have her live in my house. We were in way over our heads. I couldn't keep her safe, and I don't know the signs to look for when something like a fall happens. I'm not a nurse. We had had nurses coming in to help but often they wouldn't show up, so I had to stay up with her at night. I was losing a lot of sleep during this period.

Instead of doing more caring, as reality sunk in I pulled back and let her family put her into an assisted living facility. I didn't wallow in guilt because I finally realized that her being addicted to narcotics was too much for me to handle, and I didn't second guess my inability to take it on for any longer than the eight months that we had.

During the time that she was living with us I had twinges of guilt when I would take a break and leave a professional Caregiver with her. It felt weird to be off reading a book or even taking a nap outside in the car just to get away from the situation. That's what I was told to do in my Caregiver support group. The weirdness came from feeling so attached to her and the situation, that pulling away for a break became awkward.

I had entered the situation with the voice of another Caregiver ringing in my ear. My friend had a son with Cerebral Palsy and told me that Caregiving would be the best experience of my life as it had been for her with her son. She told me that I would have a chance to bond deeply with my mother-in-law and I approached it with that attitude at first. Now I know that every

Marian and her husband

Caregiving situation is different. Some work well and others, like mine, are very difficult.

Marian talks about feeling guilty while caring for her husband

The way I discovered that my husband had dementia was when I realized that he was no longer turning the pages of the newspaper. He was just happy to be sitting with it open on his lap. I felt guilty for not realizing what was going on at first. The guilt made me wake up to what was happening to him. In truth I had neglected to connect these changes in his behavior with any medical condition. This neglect on my part may have originated from a sense of my denial about his impending situation.

Much later we had a big commotion because after not reading the paper for months and months he had finally agreed that I could cancel the subscription but then he got upset when it no longer came. I guess I neglected to understand how attached to this lifelong routine he really was. I can't say I dwelt in feeling very guilty about this misunderstanding but I did immediately reinstate the newspaper deliveries.

As my husband's dementia progressed he would get carried away in the evenings. I never knew what would upset him. Even to this day I still expect him to come into the room and just stand there and glare at me. It would always be some crazy thing that he wanted done right then. He would accuse me of neglect and not taking care of him. Usually it was something silly like a haircut or to know what the plans were. I'd have to find some way to turn him off the subject. It was awful. Later I learned the name "sundowning" for this late-in-the-day behavior in dementia patients.

I would feel guilty that I couldn't calm his behavior down for maybe an hour, and often I would get angry or upset with him. When I would try to appear occupied with something else, it didn't work. When I would try to approach it logically, that didn't work either. If I got angry, that didn't work after a certain point. He might get distracted if he got mad back at me. I felt like I didn't handle these situations very well. I felt guilty that I didn't have a

Love stories from our hero Caregivers

solution to the problem. I had to find humor in the situation to get over the guilt. When I finally did take him for his haircut and he found out it was $16, he made a scene and said he wouldn't pay that much. I said, "Fine, just sit down and get the damn haircut."

I felt that I didn't know how to control any of it when he would get like that. Intellectually I understand that I'm not a professional but I still felt guilty that I didn't have their skills to calm him.

In terms of the decision to keep him home, I didn't think that a nursing home would prevent his falls and they would probably medicate him. Drugs have their own problems. I didn't think that I was being neglectful to keep him home with me. Once I decided I blocked out the choice to have him go to a nursing home and therefore didn't feel guilty about keeping him in our home.

I know other people who put their loved ones in homes but their situations were more serious. I don't think my husband had full blown Alzheimer's but rather dementia. Aside from the "sundowning," he was generally content. Most of his care I was able to provide so neglect wasn't really an issue. I did have help and only once did I have to call the fire department to help me lift him after he had fallen.

Musings on Mayeroff:
The focus needs to be on our caring rather than relief from our guilt feelings. By having almost lost those we care for by doing harm, losing our tempers or neglecting our duties do we in the end come to appreciate the great value the entire experience of caring has been.[53]

Author's reflections:
Sometimes it's just a matter of getting back on the right track with our caring that allows us to overcome our guilt, but the idea is not to dwell on our guilt. The idea is rather to learn from it. The takeaway here is more about appreciating the opportunities Caregiving offers us for self-awareness and growth, than in merely ridding ourselves of guilt.

How did you handle your feelings of guilt as a Caregiver?

Liz talks about breaking down while caring for her mother-in-law

If guilt is involved in my having a breakdown, that's what happened. I finally realized that I really didn't know what I was doing with my mother-in-law's care, and it was emotionally draining. In looking back I also don't know how I ended up not taking care of myself while she was living with us. I'm sure this total engagement in her care while having these feelings of inadequacy, lack of sleep and lack of any significant breaks from my Caregiving contributed to my guilt and despair.

We were given a gift certificate for my husband and I to go to dinner and I ended up sobbing and crying uncontrollably the entire time we were in the restaurant. I could not stop. This was something I had never experienced before. It felt purely emotional and when it came out, I was entirely drained. It was a real low point in the situation of our caring for my husband's mom. I felt guilty that I wasn't up to the task of taking care of this complicated woman and finally understood how it had caused me to neglect myself in many important ways that would have sustained me.

On top of the day in and day out caring for my mother-in-law, this was also during the time that my husband's sister was deciding that their mother should go to an assisted living facility. They had picked one that was far away from where we lived. I felt guilty that I didn't want to travel so far to continue to care for her, but I saw I had no choice in the matter. This all was happening about eight months into my Caregiving journey.

Marian talks about how she handled guilt while caring for her husband

Even though I had the guilt, I didn't dwell on it because I had to keep going. It did make me wonder how long I could go on Caregiving for him. The question for me was whether I was doing a good enough job and whether he was suffering more because of any lack of skills that I may have had especially around his behavioral issues. It wasn't that I felt that I was neglecting him--far from it--but rather, were my skills up to the task when he would start to act crazy?

Musings on Mayeroff:
The awareness that springs out of a feeling of guilt beckons us to reflect on ourselves and our care for the other. By overcoming a particular difficulty we can heal what's broken within ourselves and restore our caring for the other person.[54]

Author's reflections:
Guilt is a great attention getter. Because it makes us uncomfortable it grabs our focus. When we put it aside we miss the chance to heed what has gone awry in the Caregiving relationship. Feelings of guilt can dog us until we solve the problem; if left unresolved, they can haunt us irrevocably.

Reckoning with guilt over things done or gone wrong can keep us honest about our Caregiving. It nudges us to do better and to take advantage of the good things that Caregiving can bring to us when done from the heart.

What did you learn about yourself from your feelings of guilt in Caregiving?

Liz talks about seeing her mother-in-law for the real person that she was beyond her addiction

After she died I felt guilty about how I had been viewing my mother-in-law and her addiction. I didn't respect her as a person anymore. I realized I was being a very narrow and judgmental person when it came to how I was remembering her. This response probably came out of my feeling so overwhelmed and upset as her Caregiver. I don't usually see myself like this so the guilt made me take another look at the way I was viewing the situation.

It took some time but after she died I learned to separate who she truly was from her addictive behaviors. It actually took a long time to learn how to do this. It helped when I went to see Elvis Presley's museum. I had also thought of him as a loser and an addict but when I saw his body of work I was able to see his humanity. I learned to soften and do this with the memories of my mother-in-law as well. In this way I learned that I can change how I see someone and be more flexible and generous in my opinions.

Marian talks about what she learned about herself while caring for her husband

My guilt showed me that I was human. I learned that I had a breaking point and that things my husband said could make me mad. We had rarely fought during our six decades of marriage but his dementia changed all that. I learned that sometimes my problem solving skills and my ability to improvise just weren't going to be enough. I felt guilty that I wasn't super human and his dementia behavior was often a bigger problem than I could handle.

Marian talks about feeling guilty because she put her father in a mental hospital

The main thing I felt guilty about with my father was leaving him in the padded cell that first night in the mental hospital. It had taken all day after my mother suddenly handed him over to me to finally get him placed. It was a horrible guilty feeling that I had, but on the other hand, I knew he was safe. He wasn't in a room with the other mentally ill patients. He was in his own private room. I felt the guilt when I wondered with his Alzheimer's what he could grasp about what was happening to him.

What appalled me about the situation was that I needed to pull strings to get him into the hospital and into this padded cell. It was a weekend and the usual channels were closed to us. Because I had so many connections and wasn't afraid to ask for their help, I learned I could take charge of this extremely difficult situation that my mother left me in. She had given me no notice that she would be handing my father over to me on that particular day and this left me with precious little options.

At the same time I learned about myself that I could understand that my father's safety was more important than the guilt I was feeling, and that when I needed help I was able to call on others.

Chapter 19

Mutual or one-sided care for the long or the short of it

Musings on Mayeroff:
By its broadest definition, our caring doesn't need to be returned, however in a meaningful friendship the caring is mutual. Friends care for each other and in so doing become stronger as individuals. Caring on the part of one person inspires the other to return that caring.[55]

Author's reflections:
Two kinds of relationships are relevant here. There are equal-standing relationships such as good friendships and love relationships. There are also relationships of unequal status, for example those that teachers have with their students, therapists have with their clients and doctors have with their patients. Both kinds of relationships involve caring. Each person has the opportunity to flourish in their own right but for different reasons.

In an equal relationship both parties care for and nurture each other over time. This isn't a tradeoff of "if I care for you then you care for me," but an intrinsic caring in which both give freely of themselves, their commitment, their talents and their attentions to building the relationship.

When the relationship is unequal, then the growth in the person doing the caring comes when they observe that the person that they are caring for is learning and/or maturing thanks to their input or their "being there" for them.

Caring doesn't need to be a tradeoff, or a quid pro quo, as they say: if I care for you then you care for me. As we have seen, it can but doesn't have to be mutual. As a Caregiver, is your Caregiving relationship mutual or something else?

Joe M. talks about the mutual caring with his wife as they were each other's Caregivers at different times

With my wife there was no trading or keeping track when it came to our caring. We did what we had to do when we had to do it. Our caring was never one-sided. Back in the late 80's I had a heart attack and was laid up for four months. My wife took care of me then with the same love and devotion that

I had when I cared for her when she had cancer. My care for her wasn't a pay back and would have been the same regardless.

Joe M. talks about the mutual relationship he now has with his kids

Now that my kids are grown the caring has become more equal. There isn't a day that goes by that they don't call and we don't talk. We didn't drift apart when my wife died. The caring is the same as it always was, but we all have a feeling that something is missing. That shared experience has pulled us together. I don't ever see them forgetting their mother or losing the bond I have with them now.

Joe M. talks about the one-sided caring for his employees

I'm retired now, but when I had my employees, I took care of them and listened to their problems, but I didn't expect them to care for me in the same way. It was more one-sided. I accepted that because of my role as their boss. I tried to be fair and be equally concerned for all of them.

I helped them out when they had car accidents and deaths in their families by giving them time off, space to recover and making sure they were financially covered during difficult times. They were very appreciative because they each had a minimum of fifteen years with me and we were like a family.

Joe P. talks about his mutual friendship with his mentor

With my mentor and coach our caring was two-sided, especially in the later years. During all the early years of our relationship I learned so much from just being around him. I wanted to emulate how he was in the world.

As we grew closer in his later years I can't say exactly what I gave him, but I do know he appreciated and enjoyed our friendship as we grew older together. It might have been my craziness, humor, irreverence and joy of life that attracted him to me. I was his court jester. I also didn't put him on a pedestal. We were two equals who enjoyed sports. I didn't realize it at first, but he knew we were equals before I did.

As he experienced aging, he still kept his humor and talked about the changes he was going through. He would joke about how he had gone from being an Olympic marathon runner to where the kids on the street could now walk faster than him. When his health started to fail he was still active in the choices about how he wanted doctors to treat him. He remained a master of his fate. I wasn't really his Caregiver because he was so involved in setting things up for himself. Frankly I don't think anyone planned their ending better. He was aware of everything that was going on. Being a part of his process was a spiritual experience that we were able to share. At the very end of his life he only asked two people to be at his bedside, me and another friend.

During his illness I remained who I was and always remembered who he was, even though his health was failing him. I treated him the same way

I always had, including my irreverence. The caring was still mutual in most ways. As he became more frail he assigned everybody in his circle a job. My job was to accompany him to the doctor or the hospital. I would make all the arrangements for transportation and scheduling. I also let him know that if he needed me for additional help, and I could help him in any way, and that I would be there.

Musings of Mayeroff:
Some types of caring situations come to a natural end while others continue over many decades. Some types of caring situations are only successful if they end satisfactorily while others end without a formal conclusion due to changing circumstances. Some types of caring relationships need to continue so that devotion, trust and knowing each other can all deepen over time.[56]

Author's reflections:
No teacher would want their students to stay with them year after year and never graduate. No therapist would want someone to be in therapy for many years without making progress. These relationships are successful if they eventually come to a mutually positive end.

Each type of Caregiving relationship has its own timeline as caring for someone in need can fit into many time frames. Caregiving can be short term, acute care; it can take place over many years where the relationship deepens over time; or, it can be intermittent with a number of episodes of all-consuming care.

Was your Caregiving long- or short-term?

Joe M. talks about how long he cared for his wife

I took care of my wife for two and a half years after she was diagnosed with cancer. It got progressively more difficult as it went along. Somehow I found the physical strength to make it through. Now it's hard to believe I could do all that. I think that the hardest thing about my type of Caregiving was when we were anticipating that the situation would get better and it kept getting worse. There's a roller coaster of emotions that is very stressful as the situation alternates between hope and disappointment.

It was also hard to watch her suffer towards the end. I can't say I felt her pain exactly, but it felt like it was twisting inside my body and mind that this poor woman had to suffer and go through all this. In the end you almost don't want them to suffer anymore but you also don't want them to close their eyes and say goodbye for the last time either.

Joe P. talks about caring for his father over many years

My caring for my father was ongoing over many years and began when I went down to visit him and my mother in Florida after she had been diagnosed with Alzheimer's. I recognized that he needed my help. That was over 30 years ago. I would visit them in Florida 2 to 3 times a year. When I was down there I would give him breaks to go out. I would also talk with him, and stimulate him with our common interests. This level of caring for my dad lasted until my mother finally died eleven years later.

About 13 years ago things changed and I began to notice that my father was aging quickly and that I needed to become more involved in his care directly. I went down to see him every few months. He had a woman to cook for him who had started when Mom was still alive but her health started to fail so he was left alone again.

After my wife died I always kept a bag packed just in case I would need to suddenly go down to Florida to be with him. About 12 years ago, after his gall bladder surgery, he was very sick. My brother and I went down and saw that the situation was quite serious. My brother left after 3 days and I realized I couldn't leave because of my father's frailty. I ended up staying with him for over 3 months.

At the end of my stay I realized that he needed ongoing help. He could do some things to care for himself, but he couldn't do everything. That's when I hired the next door neighbor to cook and clean for him and check up on him. She was a hairdresser so she also cut his hair. She later ended up leaving her husband suddenly and went off with a new boyfriend. My father went downhill very quickly after that. He was very hurt by the situation.

My Caregiver role grew from that point on. I was constantly on the phone and went down to Florida more frequently. I made sure that the other more nearby members of our family would stop by to see him and shop for him. I finally started getting calls from his doctors suggesting that he go to a nursing home. He was just too old to live on his own.

All his life he had insisted on never wanting to go to a nursing home. I assured him that I would do whatever I had to do to keep him home. I screened all the calls I would get from the case workers who were checking on him. I assured them that he was coherent and that the house being a mess wasn't a reason to put him in a nursing home. He had two women cleaning for him and watching out for him. This stabilized the situation for a while.

His aging finally caught up with him. He was 94, had severe arthritis in his hands and was always in pain. He also had anxiety about being put in a nursing home. He needed to care for his diabetes and mostly he would. Then there started to be times when he would screw up and either forget to take his medications for his blood sugar or take too much.

We had to get him to accept services and find alternate ways for people to come in and take care of him. Finally one night I was on the phone with him for 4 hours, and that same night he died in his sleep.

Musings on Mayeroff:
Caring for another helps to make us strong.[57]

Author's reflections:
We all wonder if we will be able to rise to the occasion if called on to care for another. We want to be able to give without asking for anything back. Knowing that we are able to accomplish little miracles when called upon for another adds to our self-confidence and self-satisfaction. An inner strength develops when selflessly we don't relinquish our commitment to care. We know that we survived the worst and were able to continue to care through it all without ever looking at what we would be getting in exchange.

How have you become strengthened through your caring?

Joe M. talks about his wife giving him strength and now having difficulty finding it on his own

I was kept strong through my wife's appreciation of my caring for her. She appreciated the fact that I was there and wanted to help her. In a way we gave each other strength through the process.

Now that she is gone I no longer feel that strength. There are days I wake up with a fire in me and there are others days when I don't feel anything. An example would be that I'm trying to freshen up the house, especially the bedrooms and the hallway. Two of the bedrooms are almost done, two aren't even close and the hallway is half finished and I really don't care. When my wife was alive we would have worked on the plans together and it would have been done in a week. I would have done it and done it well and cleaned up my mess out of respect for her. Now there's no one there so I leave the mess for later. I suppose my strength came from having someone there to care for.

Right now I feel that there's more to me that's missing then that's here. I want to live for my three children and my grandchildren but there is a big hole in my heart. I'm aware that my wife is in every dream but I can't remember those dreams for the life of me.

I do feel that my wife is watching over me. Somehow she gets me to do things she wants me to do and infuses me with a strength from I don't know where.

One great example was a Sunday that I was having dinner with friends and I had taken her car. I was leaving for Florida two days later and my kids wanted me to take the Corvette that I had just taken out of storage. I was planning to drive her car. When I came out from dinner her car wouldn't start; I couldn't even turn the key and we had to have it towed. The mechanic told me he wouldn't be able to get the part we needed for several days, and a Tuesday departure for Florida was out of the question. So I took the Corvette. I know that was her doing. Driving that Corvette lifted my mood and I felt more confident on my trip.

Joe P. talks about his father's example giving him strength

My pop bolstered my strength for Caregiving because he was such a wonderful role model. When I discussed the early stages of my mom's Alzheimer's with him he matter of factly said that he was taking classes at a local community college to understand the disease better.

While my brother was suggesting that the situation would be too much for my dad and that he should put our mom in a nursing home, my dad had everything under control for their future together. He was committed to never having her go to a home as long as he could take care of her at home.

I learned from that as I took care of my own wife when she had cancer. I stayed in her room for a month and helped her as she was dying. I learned that loyalty and strength from my dad.

Chapter 20

Limits and boundaries of caring

Musings on Mayeroff:
Caring can only take place when two individuals recognize and respect their separate identities.[58]

Author's reflections:
While on the surface a relationship may appear to be one of caring, unless there is mutual respect and both partners maintain their individuality, true caring will not mature. In the extreme, neglect or abuse may even arise.

Caregivers first need to know their own limits, what they can handle and how to recharge their energies. They must learn what their needs are and include them in the overall care plan. When Caregivers go beyond their limits they can experience frustration, lose their patience and finally "burn out" with feeling overwhelmed.

Each of us has an emotional boundary that keeps us intact as a person. When the boundary between two people which protects their individuality is breached, the relationship becomes troubled. One example of this breach is called a "morbid dependency," or when one person feels they cannot survive without the other. Another example, "malevolent manipulation," arises when one person controls the other in order to meet their own needs. Or, in an "overprotected relationship," one person prevents the other from fully experiencing life due to their own excessive fears of harm being done them.[59]

When two people in a relationship have fully developed personalities and well-defined personal boundaries and the Caregiver understands their limits, it allows each of them to think and act independently, the potential is there for optimal Caregiving.

Have you ever tried to exceed your boundaries to manipulate situations or your loved one? Do you know of others who have?

Sarah talks about unhealthy relationships in her Caregiver support group

There were several examples of couples in the group where the care recipient was the controlling and manipulative one in the relationship. They would overstep their boundaries with a goal of controlling their Caregiver. They didn't want them to go out, have their own friends or their own life. Because they were in this manipulative role they would insist that their Caregiver sit on the couch and watch TV with them, but meanwhile they would be asleep within minutes. They demanded this excessive devotion and time from their Caregivers. They didn't seem to understand that their Caregiver may need to get away so they could be replenished and recharged. The care recipient didn't connect that taking time away would also help the Caregiver to ultimately be more available once they were rested. Caregiving in this context can be very similar to abuse in other types of relationships.

One person in the support group had barely known her new partner before she had been diagnosed with cancer. Once things changed she became entirely devoted as a Caregiver and lost much of herself and her own former life in the process. Because there hadn't been a long term relationship previous to the onset of the illness it seemed more obvious to the group that she was acting like a martyr. For her this excessive devotion became almost a total dependency on the situation. She hadn't set limits to her care and as a result the more that was asked the more she would give with no end in sight. Boundaries between the two were being lost and her identity was being dissolved.

As I listened to these stories I thought that one solution to prevent these extremes might be to form a care team so that the Primary Caregiver has resources to draw on, be it friends, family or community members who divide various chores amongst themselves. That way everyone would have time away and no one would be totally responsible for keeping everything running smoothly. That feeling of never being able to get away from Caregiving is very hard. So is the extra worry about one's own health and fearing what would happen if their health as a Caregiver were to fail. There would also be more eyes to witness and prevent the onset of abusive or destructive relationships within the Caregiving.

Suzanne talks about independence and setting limits as a Caregiver for her husband

Becoming my husband's nurse was outside of anything I would have imagined I, a Family Caregiver, would have to do. I learned what I needed to do and did it without manipulation or overprotection. He was physically dependent on me towards the end but I didn't abuse it, and he retained his independence in his decisions and attitudes.

I did have the expenses of our business together and no one was there to keep it going. We had rent and everything else that goes along with having an office. To keep all that going by myself while my husband was sick felt like it was beyond what I could do as a Caregiver. I had reached my limits and finally had to shut things down.

In general during our long marriage I never tried to manipulate my husband to do anything he didn't want to do. I never had to.

Have you been overprotective of your loved one? What happened to your boundaries?

Suzanne talks about her feelings of being overprotective with her husband

I felt that I was overprotective at times as my husband's health deteriorated. Ironically as I look back I now think that at first I hadn't been protective enough and had trusted the doctors too much. Once I stepped up my husband didn't realize it because it was behind the scenes as I intervened with the medical staff. It was the first time I didn't consult him and was doing something without his knowledge. In my judgment the boundaries of who he was were being put aside for a higher good.

When I finally spoke up to his doctor about what I considered negligence and fired him, my husband didn't know I had done that. I wanted to protect him from the negative emotions so he could focus on getting better. Usually my husband was in on all the decisions about his health but in this instance I took over and did what I had to do. I may have overstepped my boundaries but it was in the name of supporting him in getting better. I wasn't disrespecting him. I can imagine when overprotection might be harmful. As a teacher I saw parents who were overly protective of their children but in Caregiving there are times when the person needs an advocate to stand in for them.

Sarah talks about being overprotective with her mom

I felt hyper-vigilant about my mom's health not so much overprotective. Since the disease was progressing faster than I could keep up with it, I would always be afraid of what would happen next. I was running down information and programs as fast as I could but I was having trouble keeping up. I became totally involved in her care. At first I had respectful boundaries with her but the demands of the illness weakened them as I became more involved. I was trying to anticipate my mother's needs and leading the efforts to get her services. She was less involved in this process and certainly wasn't the initiator. I wasn't following her lead but rather trying desperately to stay ahead of her illness.

My limits as a Caregiver became the rapid progression of the cancer. It was a race. The things I thought I could control, like applying for Access-a-Ride, ended up not being helpful because she could no longer go out by the time the application was processed. Same thing when I ordered her wheelchair because by then she was bedridden.

I'm familiar with the fact that hyper-vigilance is also a part of the experience of trauma so in a way I see I was probably being slowly traumatized by the situation. It was hard to feel proud of my extra efforts when I could see I was too late but looking back I see that I had done the best I could at the time even if I was overstepping my boundaries with my mother.

Author's reflections:
A Caregiver may begin to perceive their loved one becoming increasingly dependent on them. Rather than being alarmed, or even feeling uncomfortable about it, some Caregivers look for ways to maintain this dependency. They may be fulfilling a need to be wanted or to feel important, but such a relationship is ultimately dysfunctional.

In order for the person being cared for to thrive, their interpersonal boundaries need to be clear and their autonomy viable. Encouraging dependency restricts their ability to fully experience their own lives.

The same is true for the Caregiver. Becoming defined by their dependency on a need to be indispensable to another can damage their own functioning and wellbeing.

Can you do things independently of the person you are caring for?

Suzanne talks about needing to stay with her husband in the hospital

During the last five months of my husband's life I was at the hospital every day and so was my daughter. Sometimes she would go back home for less than a day to take care of her affairs and then come right back. Even though my husband was emotionally dependent on us to be there, he still was autonomous and made all his own decisions. I didn't change my manner with my husband. I always showed him respect for who he was and encouraged him to be himself. As a result he was hopeful until the end that he would somehow beat these health issues and we would all go back to our lives.

I suppose to an extent I was dependent on my role as Caregiver. It was hard for me to get away from it even for a short while. I would try to go to some events and meetings but it was hard to arrange. I'm involved with a transplant group as their secretary. I did manage to get to one meeting but this was because my daughter was able to be there with my husband in the hospital. I was able to go to a few things if I really had something I needed to do. I could arrange it because my daughter would be there. An example would be that occasionally I was able to leave the hospital to get my hair done.

Sarah talks about the difficulties of being able to leave her mother

It was very difficult for me to leave my mother during her illness. I did go on vacation for about 10 days, but I had to call in from Canada. I was also quite preoccupied with worry while I was there. I had my son and my partner with me on the trip, but I was always aware that I might get called back if something important happened to my mother while we were away. I was the one who became dependent on the situation. I had lost myself a bit during this time, especially in my reduced ability to enjoy a social life.

Sarah talks about a member of the support group finding her independence

One of the group members owned a house with her lover and when she got sick and could no longer climb stairs they had to have separate bedrooms. The Caregiver felt guilty that she liked having her own space in the house. She needed her boundaries and some time alone. There were hints that maybe they wouldn't stay together when her partner got stronger, but she didn't want to do anything about it now while she was still needed. She loved having the time and space to be alone and away from her role as a Caregiver. This feeling was similar to the topic discussed in the Virginia Wolf book, **A Room of One's Own.**

Author's reflections:
Caregivers perform so many tasks for their loved ones that it is difficult even to keep track of them, and so it is easy to exceed the Caregiver's limits of what they can handle. Caregivers run the risk of "burnout" and being overwhelmed. As a result, Caregivers will generally admit to lost tempers, irritation, sarcasm and sometimes physical abuse. It is especially difficult to take on so much when the person they are caring for isn't able to be appreciative, either due to their illness or due to a kind of self-involvement that often accompanies illness. If Caregivers are appreciated at all it is often not about each sock that they fold but more for the overall care that they are able to give.

When a Caregiver sets the stage for the ability of the care recipient to maintain their dignity through difficult times, they are often also setting the stage for positive outcomes in their Caregiving and for themselves. They may not receive the recognition they deserve for each accomplishment, but hopefully they are recognized for their ability to create a caring and supportive environment for the both of them.

How does appreciation of your efforts affect your Caregiving?

Suzanne talks about her husband's implied appreciation

Because of how well I knew my husband, I know he was generally appreciative of my care. He didn't say it but I knew intuitively. I don't know how he would have been if I or my daughter hadn't been there. I feel that our care allowed my husband to continue to hope for the best outcomes even when things got tough. I always made sure to consider his personality and feelings so that the dignity that he maintained throughout his life remained intact.

I am proud of the care I showed my husband and only felt limited by the medical care he was receiving. I would have liked to have been able to change things before they became so out of control for all of us. Instead of growth and comfort his medical care destroyed him. I felt limited by the lack of timely information I had received. I know my husband appreciated what we did for him but he had no idea of the real truth of what had happened to him. Had I known what I needed to know to make good decisions early on, I feel that my husband might still be with us.

Sarah talks about appreciation in her life and her support groups

I don't think you can wait for something positive to come out of every act of kindness. But since I haven't been in that situation on the receiving end I don't really know how much appreciation I would show. Maybe if it was entirely a one sided relationship I would appreciate small efforts from my Caregiver. When I am the Caregiver I prefer appreciation, but I don't expect it and know I won't always get it. Appreciation would definitely help the situation in terms of being able to continue at a high level of Caregiving without getting overwhelmed or discouraged.

In the Caregivers I have worked with, if the disease isn't terminal there is a tremendous thrust towards returning to some kind of normalcy. The idea is to return to work and a social life as soon as possible. Maybe this is the growth out of the situation for both people.

Sarah talks about her mother's dignity

In terms of the big picture with taking care of my mother, I don't know if I was thinking of it as her dignity. I wanted her to have her autonomy so she wouldn't be pushed around. I wanted her to have control over her decision making and that it was up to me to accept what she wanted. For example she ended up not wanting chemotherapy. I read about what it would have been in her case and it just didn't make any sense anyway. Regardless I still would have left it up to her to make that call.

My mother wasn't the type to express her appreciation so I had to go on a feeling I had that she might be grateful for my efforts. I still would have liked a deathbed reconciliation of some sort. Maybe I do long for her appreciation of my Caregiving too.

Family Caregiving is a difficult task and, although no one can be perfect at it, many hold up perfection as their goal. Having a bad day is normal for Caregivers during an experience that can resemble a rollercoaster ride. Bumping up against their limits is a common experience for many Caregivers and becomes a frequent test of their skill, generosity and devotion. In a way they are getting to know themselves in a deep way that the average life doesn't offer.

In addition, some Caregivers need motivation to spark them to do the best they possibly can in good times and bad. Wanting to feel proud of a job well done is one way to motivate a Caregiver. No Caregiver is proud of those times when they lost their temper or became abusive. In order to avoid such unenlightened behavior, an out of control Caregiver will need to seek out professional help and attend to their own physical and emotional health needs.

Does your Caregiving ever feel like a rollercoaster?

Suzanne talks about ups and downs with her husband

My family had ups and downs especially right before my husband's death. During the last five months of his life there were times he could come home from the hospital and that was an up and then he'd have to go right back again which was a downer. He was home very little because he ended up in three hospitals and rehabilitation facilities during those five months. I felt that he was discharged too soon from the one hospital. In that case I especially felt they were trying to get everyone out of that hospital for Christmas Eve. He ended up having to go back two days later. During this time we mostly had our emotional downs to deal with due to the medical issues he was facing. The circumstances made it hard to stay upbeat and hopeful.

    I stayed by him during this whole time even though sometimes I knew I was near my limits as a human being. It wasn't so much about my being perfect but I was proud of the things I was able to accomplish as a Caregiver. I tried to do little things like make his favorite foods. When he was home we tried to make him as comfortable as possible.

    At two points we did have the visiting nurse service come to the house and they were very good. It was great to have this outside support. My daughter and I had to give him intravenous antibiotics three times a day when the nurses weren't there. I had never done that before so the nurses checked that we were doing it right. We were determined that nothing bad would happen on our watch. This was part of our growth and a reason to feel proud.

    I needed to push beyond my familiar limits and develop the skills of a nurse. I suppose this was an up in a back door sort of way. I am proud that my daughter and I could handle all this. So yes, I think this emotional rollercoaster is common for Caregivers, but I see that each circumstance is unique.

Sarah talks about the ups and downs caring for her own mom

While I was taking care of my mom my moods would be up and down. I would go from being depressed to thinking a lot about what cancer is, and then there was the fear. I would want to go and have myself checked out. The fear was almost contagious by just being in the situation of watching what cancer was doing even though my mother accepted the fact that she had been a smoker and now had lung cancer. She was more logical. It made sense to her that smoking caused her cancer and in fact her making this connection caused her to stop smoking for the last 14 months of her life. I, however, was left with the fear of witnessing her failing health and the illogical fear that I myself would get cancer too just by seeing what her cancer was doing to her. The whole situation would bring me down and I had a limited ability to cheer myself up in the face of these fears.

    Another aspect that was a downer was that I would have liked to have had a sort of saying goodbye with my mother but that never happened. She didn't say much to show that she appreciated what I was doing to help her. Only once did she give me a back-handed compliment to thank me by saying, "Considering how we feel about each other it is nice that you have done this for me." I would have felt better and maybe more proud of myself as her Caregiver if we had been able to be closer as people.

I would have ups when I would think of the problems I had solved with my persistence, even though these successes weren't acknowledged by my mother. For example she hated the doctor I found and she hated the hospital, but no matter I still felt proud of completing the project to get her there. I felt generally proud of myself that ultimately I had her health and her best interests at heart and was left with a feeling of competence afterwards. The situation defined more sharply who my mother was, who I was, and I got to see my heart at work. In the end I was left with a good feeling.

Section D

Focus on caring for people

Chapter 21

Being connected by our caring for others

Musings on Mayeroff:
In all types of relationships we enter another person's world. We are able to see their world the way they do. We know deeply how they feel about their lives, what they are striving to become and what they need in order to thrive.[60]

Author's reflections:
With careful attention we can "walk a mile in another's shoes" with people experiencing lives very different from our own. With children with autism and people who show signs of dementia, for example, it would seem impossible to enter their world, but it can be done within certain limits when we make the effort to connect. Someone who can connect intrinsically with another person is able to have a deep understanding of their reality, of seeing, even as out of their eyes.

Cultivating a deep understanding of another is a type of symbiosis that breaks down the boundaries that keep us separate. This can have positive effects when we enter another's world.

Caring can offer specific challenges to our ability to connect. When caring for someone with Alzheimer's disease for example we enter their often distorted world. Therapeutic lying has been described as an uncontested going along with what the Alzheimer's patient is saying, no matter how farfetched or implausible it may be, unless their safety is involved.

Caregivers often find this acquiescence helps to minimize stress in the person in their care. It also allows for a deeper connection to someone with such an altered reality. The use of therapeutic lies comes out of the understanding we have of the person's experience and tailoring our truths to fit theirs. These "lies" can become part of the conversation, based on the Caregiver's understanding of the cognitive failings of the patient. Going along with how they are seeing the world allows us to share in their version of reality.

When a Caregiver makes the difficult adjustment of sidelining the "real" in order to connect to another's version of the world, we then see how meaningful and challenging caring can be.

Are you able to enter the world of the person you are caring for and really know how they feel, what will nourish them and their goals?

Barb talks about how she developed her caring skills

I learned more about how to feel for others when as a child I volunteered as a candy striper in the hospital. I learned how to listen to others, understand the world from their perspective and I also learned how to discover what their goals and dreams were. I had forgotten about that volunteer experience until my sister-in-law reminded me that she had worked at the same hospital. As I performed my volunteer duties I was able to see more and more of what people needed and how I could be of service. I would listen to them and try to put myself in their shoes whenever I could. Sometimes just listening was enough to see them start to feel better about their situation. I really enjoyed the experience.

At sixteen I volunteered in a psychiatric hospital. Later I worked on a team for several years in college with an child who had autism. We all learned a lot about what goes on in the mind of someone affected by autism. I started to see the world in a different way because of this child and my attempting to learn what they needed without a word being said.

Looking back I think I always had a Caregiver's soul and the ability to get inside what someone else is feeling. I've had an ability to pick up on other people's emotions and could mirror back to them or help them reflect on their situation. It is easy to put myself in their world and know what they are going through. I was always a good listener. Once I discovered what they needed I could see how to help them with their goals and direction. It's hard to teach that. It's more about who you are as a caring person. I was drawn to these different experiences early on and that helped me develop my skills even more. Being connected to and serving others has been my lifelong ambition.

Toni talks generally about people

I know that often people feel very strongly about things and they aren't always able to express themselves. I try to get to know what a person needs to reach their highest goals so that if there's anything I can do to make their journey easier, that's what I do.

In my experience they might have dreams and I would never want to be the cause of them losing their dreams. That would be terrible. It's almost like losing your life when you lose a dream. If I am connected to another person and really care about them then I'll make this kind of effort to get to know more about them and their dreams.

Musings on Mayeroff:
The person being cared for can find comfort knowing they are not alone in tough times, when there is someone standing next to them who can relate to their situation, someone who knows them intimately and, with this knowledge, can help them overcome obstacles.[61]

Author's reflections:
Our minds sometimes play funny tricks on us, seeking out the negative, even about ourselves. When illness or challenges interfere in our lives going through these difficult times alone can accentuate this gloom, and before you know it the world looks like a dark, scary place. Having someone to remind us of our strengths and our value can lower the volume on our oftentimes critical inner voices. Caregivers often are the outer voices of comfort and strength that drown out the inner voices of doubt and negativity.

Do you think that the person you are caring for is comforted by your knowing them intimately?

Barb talks about how she relates to her mother

My mother certainly knows and understands that I am able to relate to her and her situation. She feels my love as being authentic because it is demonstrated to her in many ways, my calling, caring about her, visiting when I can. She feels it the most when I am actually there with her and we spend time hugging because that's what shows her my feelings the most clearly.

I appreciate who she is at 93 even though most people think she is much younger. I neither build her up to be someone she isn't nor do I underestimate her powers. There are so many stereotypes about older adults it is really important to get to know each person as an individual the way I have with my mom. She still surprises me and I continue to grow in my understanding of who she is. She likes to tell people her age to see the look of surprise on their faces. I hope she's as lively at 105. The doctor said she could live to be 115.

I see her both for who she is and who she has been. Out of respect for how well I know her and her dignity I don't try to insist that she have more help than she needs. I think she appreciates that I am not overbearing and can see who she truly is as a spirited woman in her community.

Toni talks about the difficulties of relating to her brother's situation

At first I wasn't good at relating to what my brother was going through. When the doctors gave him three or six months to live, he would tell me. Instead of validating his feelings of fear or worry I would ask him why he was listening to the doctors. I would remind him that in the old days they wouldn't have had these tests to tell him he has all these things wrong and he probably would have been fine.

I'm healthy and my life isn't on the line. One day I might be sick and then maybe I'll understand his perspective more. Without that it's easy to say how I would be in his situation but I haven't experienced it yet. It is hard to stay connected to him emotionally when I don't share the same fears and pressures in my own life.

When I finally realized that he's probably really terrified I started listening to the emotion in what he was saying. Now I listen to him more and I can understand that this is his perspective. He doesn't have to share my perspective. Our relationship has gotten closer as a result of my being more open to his views of things.

Author's reflections:
We have a choice about how involved with other people we want to become. This can apply to our families, social groups, the houses of worship we attend or our work lives. Yes, we often have other people around us, but it is up to us how connected—or close—to them we will be.

Symbiotic relationships involve getting in the trenches with another. We merge our identities and emotions. Empathy allows us to connect to someone else's experience without taking on the experience itself. Empathy helps me understand your fear and why you would be afraid without taking on the fear myself. A Veteran soldier can listen to the recent experiences of the soldier in combat without needing to get back in the trenches with them.

In a broader sense some of us feel deeply connected to the communities in which we live, the organizations to which we belong, the schools we have attended, and our spiritual communities. We care deeply about the day-to-day activities of the group and may be willing to give of ourselves as officers or committee members. Others of us feel comfortable looking more from a distance at the formal and informal groups to which we belong. It may feel safer that way.

This choice of how connected we want to become applies to our Caregiving. We can provide care without really making any deep emotional connection to the person we are assisting. We may choose to remain emotionally distant due to a fear that we are giving up too much of ourselves or taking on too much of their experience as our own.

Being close to another person, especially one in great need of us, cannot help but be affecting. It asks us to strike a very delicate balance between maintaining our autonomy and sense of self with losing our sense of self in, or merging with, the other person in their need. This is the darker side of symbiosis when we get lost in our connection to another person. When this happens in a Caregiving setting, ultimately the quality of care and ability to make sound decisions suffer.

True caring more involves empathy. Empathy is the ability to put oneself in another's shoes without getting lost ourselves. When another person is sad or angry, for example, empathy comes into play if we can understand how it feels to that person without becoming sad or angry ourselves. It is a skill that needs to be cultivated. Sometimes we choose not to get involved with another person and their problems because we fear that we will start taking on the emotions of that person as our own. We fear that their depression or frustration, whatever their troubles, will become ours.

How do the feelings and behavior of the person you are caring for affect you?

Barb talks about how her mother is reacting after her father's death

My mother has grown into an amazing person since his my father's death. We are more like friends now. I just got back from spending a week with her in Florida. Our relationship has become warm and very personal.

My Caregiving consists of being sensitive to where my mom is emotionally. I've watched her blossom from the loss of my dad into a caring person. A good friend of hers had just lost her spouse and my mom was able to be her Caregiver because of what she went through with losing my dad. She's always been very organized but now I could watch her help her friend who was completely overwhelmed by her husband's death. I saw a side of her that is very sensitive as she told her friend what she had to do by breaking down the tasks and helping her organize her papers.

Watching her recover from the loss of my dad in such a positive way makes me very proud to be her daughter. It also means that I haven't gotten lost in her sadness because I can see she is handling things very well. It has allowed us to become more than just mother and daughter in our relationship. We support each other yet we are both full people in our own lives.

Toni talks about connecting to her father

When my mother got sick with early-onset Alzheimer's the relationship with my father changed from our being argumentative to forming a team to help my mother. His reaction to what was happening with my mom was to hold on to the idea that we were a family and would somehow get through this together.

I joined him in this way of dealing with everything. We did our decision making together. He counted on me to help him make these decisions and I trusted him to never second guess me or say I was wrong after the fact. I could relate to his emotions but I didn't get lost in them. I didn't feel like we were blended into one person while we cared for my mom. We brought different things to the table. We became a team of two individuals with the same goals.

Toni talks about connecting to her brother as he experienced his mother's early onset Alzheimer's from a distance

I connected to my brother's reactions during the time we were caring for our mother because I could almost feel his pain. In a way I became his Caregiver too. He was having a lot of trouble watching our mother change so drastically. It felt like it was blowing my heart open with sadness to see how he was handling things. I did get very involved in his emotional life. I didn't know what to do to comfort him. I didn't know how to take away his pain or his fear. I would run up to see him every weekend or spend three-day weekends with him.

I wanted him to know that he was important even though he wasn't involved directly in my mom's care. When push came to shove I was there for him, even though I hadn't always been there in the past.

I was always telling him that he was "the victor" because that was his name. I would tell him he was the fighter and the winner and go do it! My efforts were all focused on improving his attitude and helping him feel strong during the suffering we were all feeling at gradually losing our mother.

Musings on Mayeroff:
Caring precludes judging one another.[62]

Author's reflections:
Judgments and preconceived notions get in the way of caring and connection. No one likes criticism from others. Some Caregivers might especially have trouble with judgmental care receivers because they may feel that they have been giving so much and are underappreciated for it.

Ours is not to judge another either. When we become Caregivers the needs and vulnerabilities of the person we are now caring for call on us to dissolve our previous judgments about their abilities, fitness levels, self-sufficiency, roles and emotional strength. As we experience new situations in our Caregiving role, we are invited to create new ideas to go along with this new path we are on.

This parent may no longer be able to care for us as our roles reverse. This athlete may no longer be able to play sports due to accident or injury. This sibling may not be able to follow the doctor's orders due to lack of motivation or lack of understanding the consequences. This husband may no longer be the strength of the family or be able to make decisions anymore about finances or plans for the future. Holding on to our old ideas or clinging to our former beliefs about them keeps us locked up emotionally and can destine us to a rough road ahead.

Have you become judgmental of the person you are caring for? If so, how has that affected your Caregiving?

Barb talks about judging her mother's living situation

I worry because I see my mother becoming more frail as she ages. I do feel that she is physically more vulnerable because of her age. Her age affects her in other ways as well.

I don't know how great it is for her to be living with so many seniors. I am judgmental about that. She is living in a place where everywhere you look there are notices that people have died, at temple, at the condominium, friend's spouses who have died. I feel that it gives the residents the idea that you are here on the earth but you don't know for how long. I can see this might just be how I see the situation and maybe she sees it differently. One way she deals with the death notices is to turn towards life in the enjoyment she finds in her grandchildren. They feed her soul. She is always getting photos of the little ones that she can enjoy. So maybe I shouldn't get involved as an outsider in this.

Musings on Mayeroff:
In our praise of the other person we convey that they are supported and admired.[63]

Author's reflections:
All too often we can tell a third party how wonderful someone is but it gets more difficult to praise the person we care for directly. When we are able to directly acknowledge another's strengths and virtues we connect deeply with them. They feel they have been seen by us and we then let them know what we admire about them. By feeling our support they are better able to achieve their goals.

Is it easy for you to praise those you care about? How do you show them you care?

Toni talks about being able to praise her brother

My greatest gift is seeing the good in others and letting them know. My brother had been a great athlete all his life until he lost his balance and could no longer see out of one eye. When he started getting sick he kept on getting headaches and couldn't do anything physical anymore.

During this time I told him a dream I had that in a past life he was a Spartan, a warrior. In my dream he won the contest, he was the victor. I told him he is a fighter and that just like his name Victor he would make it through, as long as he stopped whining. He would make it through because he has warrior blood.

I reminded him that he had overcome sickness before. I added "when others paint a bleak picture of your future they don't know you are a warrior. Life is magical." We talked about the fact that he might not make it but I said "if you survive this you want to be as strong as you can be." I suggested we set up for the negative but keep looking at the positive steps he could take.

In response to my building him up, he now can tell me that he had a great day without any qualifications. He has millions of friends who love him and even though his dreams of being a great basketball player aren't perfect he's happy. I can see it in his smile and I tell him what I see. We are closer now then we have ever been because we shared his recovery. This is how I am able to care for him.

Author's reflections:
Can we be happy for someone who gets into a better school, has a better job, finds a successful partner, wins the game or appears to "have it all"?

In this competitive world of ours we have been trained to win, to be the best at everything we do and to think badly of our competition and treat them as our enemies. The media fans the flames of this way of looking at the world.

When the person you are caring for has good things happen to them how do you react? Does it bring you closer or create separation?

Barb talks about when good things happen for her mother

I think it's great when good things happen for my mom. A few years ago she was woman of the year for Hadassah and we all went to the luncheon. She's always getting special service buttons at her job. I love to share her successes with her when she gets these kinds of recognition. It makes me feel closer to her to share her excitement and pride.

Toni talks about sharing in the successes of her brother

I'm thrilled and excited when good things happen to my brother. I also feel relieved. My heart feels a song. I know that there was a reason for his struggle and that he's going to be able to climb mountains. He's like Sisyphus. He'll climb the mountain and fall back and then climb it again. He'll eventually be able to fly but he'll have to change his behavior. He'll have to hold life differently than he used to.

When we were caring for my mother he was more of a negative, self-centered person. He's changed and can now see the goodness in the small things in life. I love watching him grow into new realizations and the hope for his future development allows me to feel more connected to him. It feels like we are on similar paths of discovery.

Musings on Mayeroff:
By acknowledging the other person they feel encouraged to be themselves. Our trusting them allows them to trust themselves and feel deserving of our trust.[64]

Author's reflections:
When comic actors or standup comedians talk about their childhood they often discuss the attention that they received for creating funny characters or making people laugh. It feels good to have others acknowledge us.

When we receive honest encouragement from others it causes our own inner critic to start to fade and we begin to feel worthy of the attention of others. In giving this same acknowledgment to others we, too, are overriding their inner critic and helping them.

How does the person you are caring for respond to your trust and acknowledgment? How does this help you to stay connected to them?

Barb talks about her mother's response to her trust and acknowledgement

We have a wonderful relationship and it is easy for us to support each other. She calls sometimes just to hear my voice. That indicates to me that she trusts me to love and listen to her. She does the same in supporting me so that makes it a very easy relationship for both of us.

Toni talks about trust in her relationships

My brother thinks that I am his hero. My father said the same thing to me when he was alive and so did my friend. I'm not sure why. I think that they all trusted me. What my brother says is that I am solid and always there for him. Generally speaking I won't let people crash and burn because I understand that on some level they are me and I am them. This is how we are connected.

Chapter 22
Caring for myself

Author's reflections:
Of course there are those folks, and we all have met at least one, who are obsessed with themselves and oblivious to the needs of others. Often these people aren't aware that there is any other way to be. They seem content with the way they are, unaware of how negatively this self-involvement may be perceived by those around them.

Often this self-centeredness stems from the lack of positive reinforcement and attention in their earlier years. Most may be incapable of becoming more self-aware or working towards personal growth and will only change if faced with profound adversity or trauma. Often, they can continue to avoid addressing their problems by surrounding themselves with people who will not challenge them or their self-image. A good number of celebrities in the fashion and entertainment industries would seem to fall into this category.

Most of us, in contrast, would be dismayed to know we are thought of as self-centered and untouched by others' needs. Having a friend call us selfish would be one of the worst things we could hear. Many Caregivers would rather sacrifice their own health and well-being in order to prove to themselves how much they care about others by putting the other's needs first.

Do you care what others think about you? Would you worry if others thought you were being selfish?

Sheri talks generally about being thought of as selfish in her relationships

In my relationships I pick people who wouldn't think badly of me. I judge myself harshly already so other people are usually kinder to me than I am to myself. If they did have a problem with me or think I am selfish, we would communicate and work it out. I care about misunderstandings. If there is something true in what they are concerned with, I am happy to apologize and I would attempt to understand their point of view.

Sheri talks about growing into her generosity over time

I've changed a lot as an adult. I have grown into a caring person who doesn't mind doing the cooking and cleaning for my partner. I now consider myself generous and aware of the needs of others.

When I was a kid I didn't do things around the house like the dishes. That wasn't my job or I hadn't thought to do them when I was younger. It wasn't because I was being selfish but that I just wasn't aware that I could offer to do them. It seems like a small issue but now when we have family gatherings they make a big deal that I'm finally doing the dishes. The teasing was fine at first but they are still making a fuss about it years later.

The real issue is that they can't see that I've grown and have become more conscious of how I can contribute. It used to bother me that they still thought I was the same as when I was a child, but now I usually just let it go. I didn't start doing the dishes for the acceptance of my family. I just do them when I want to offer that as a thoughtful gesture. It stems from the new awareness I now have as an adult about how to help out in these family situations the way I do at home and with my friends.

As a Caregiver what do you imagine those under your care think about you? For example do they appreciate your generosity or maybe think you are self-centered when you tend to your own needs?

Alicia talks about what her mother thought about her care

I know my mother was embarrassed to need my help. She was embarrassed that she could no longer take care of herself and that she had to depend on other people. She was the one who was more self-absorbed with her physical struggles. Generally speaking I think that she was happy to have me there and thankful for my generosity. I would like to think that I helped her through the dying process.

She never told me directly about what she thought about my moving down to live with her for three months. I did get a small clue however. One time, before she was bedridden, we were together in the bathroom. She did say thank you to me for taking care of her. I responded by telling her that she probably had no idea how much I loved her and that I would do anything I could for her. With that she kissed me on the nose. I was actually tending to my own needs as well as hers when I decided to live with her, but after this brief incident I think she strongly knew that it was also because I loved her.

Sheri talks about pulling back her care from her neighbor

I'm pretty sure that my neighbor thought I was being selfish during her last days before her suicide. For many years before this sad ending I know she thought that I was a very trusted friend. My friend would get involved in her substance abuse and then call from the police station on a Sunday. I went to pick her up once or twice, but I saw there wasn't going to be any change in her behavior so I had to tell her I couldn't do it anymore. That was one of the hardest things I've ever had to do in my entire life, especially knowing that she took her own life in the end.

I think she was very hurt once I decided I had to detach from her. Her situation with her addiction was seriously bringing me down. I understood how disappointed in me she felt but I just couldn't be there for her anymore.

I considered her situation but found it untenable. She wasn't prepared to change or help herself out of her troubles. I'm not a very co-dependent person anymore. I had been in a situation in my twenties where I got involved with someone I wanted to "fix" and it wasn't healthy. My approach now feels like healthy boundaries to me, not selfishness.

Musings on Mayeroff:
Since generally speaking we relate to others in a similar way to the way we relate to ourselves, we need to be able to relate our own need for self-awareness to the same needs in another.[65]

Author's reflections:
We have a tendency to see the world through our own eyes and then make judgments according to our own experiences. For example, if we have been harsh or impatient with ourselves, then that is what we may ultimately bring to others, especially when we are stressed.

On the other hand, if I am self-aware, then I can share the more supportive parts of myself with others and there is something solid to hold onto when the waters get rough. Emotional growth and self-awareness gives us built-in resiliency.

How do you balance your need for self-care with the need to care for others?

Alicia talks about balancing her needs with those of her family

I'm not always balanced when I'm on a mission. This can be when I care for someone else or even when I need to care for myself. An example is the way I committed myself to another when I went down to care for my mom for three months in Puerto Rico. I needed to completely devote myself to her and her health. That was my priority and I cancelled everything else, even caring for myself.

Creating a home for myself and my husband that's comfortable and nurturing is now my priority. In terms of making this a priority, I realized this week that the most important thing for me right now is to create a nest for myself. This is our second move in a short period of time and I really need to create a comfortable home for myself with my husband. What this means during the holidays is saying no to my family when we are invited to their gatherings and telling them that we need time alone to organize our new home. That is a bigger and more important goal this year than celebrating the holidays. I could give this level of devotion to my mother when she was dying and now I need to give the same level of devotion to myself.

Sheri talks about how much she gives in her caring

My partner isn't needy at all. It's about me being a very giving person that I have to pay attention to because I used to forget myself in the mix. My partner has some health issues and I have learned to let her take responsibility for how she is going to manage these issues. It is sometimes hard to hold back and watch her do things that cause her pain.

I have my art, music and dog to give my time to, so I've learned to only give to her when I want to give. She doesn't pressure me. It's a beautiful thing. I've had to work on my end of this over the last ten years and I have definitely grown in the process.

Musings on Mayeroff:
If we don't act on our own instinct to grow, we'll soon find ourselves incapable of understanding others' needs and shortcomings.[66]

Author's reflections:
I can only imagine in others what I have experienced myself on some level. I may not be on the exact same path as another, but we can share an understanding that we both need to grow and learn about ourselves and our purpose. If I am stagnant then another's growth can be threatening, strange or seem trivial.

Are you learning from your Caregiving or merely surviving it?

Alicia talks about learning as she cared for her mom

During the time I took care of my mom I learned a lot about my own strength. I learned a lot about myself as a person and that I can handle anything that comes my way. Things may throw me into a corner for a few days but once I get my head back in order I know what I need to do and get it done.

Caring showed me that as long as I could keep my head in the right place, I could deal with anything. I learned a lot about courage and strength and who I was as a person. I could put aside all the pain with my mom and just be there, to love and be loved.

Sheri talks about learning from all her caring

My days of merely surviving my Caregiving are long gone. I can see how much I have learned and grown with the Caregiving I have already done, even when it ended badly as in the case of my neighbor's suicide.

I say that but I still have both of my parents. They are in Las Vegas with my brother and his wife, who will mostly care for my parents when the time comes. We'll see what happens as I attempt to also care for them from a distance with frequent visits. I do think I'm beyond just going into survival mode in my Caregiving. Working on having better boundaries has certainly helped me with this and I look forward to learning more about myself and about life as I care for my parents.

Musings on Mayeroff:
Being unable to care about anything outside of ourselves inhibits our ability to truly care about ourselves. Our purpose and direction in that caring for something other than ourselves enables us to grow emotionally and spiritually. Life's fulfillment comes from service to others and our engagement in our projects, our art, and our ideas, as long as these are separate from ourselves.[67]

Author's reflections:
It would be almost impossible to care about ourselves if we weren't capable of caring about others. Since a core human need is to connect with others, when left unfulfilled we are emptied of purpose. To truly care about ourselves and to meet our need to have a purpose, we must find someone or some interest to care about deeply.

How does caring for others relate to your ability to care for yourself?

Alicia talks about her students in her Yoga classes

When my students come to class to relax I make recommendations about how they should take time to relax at home. I give them what I think is good advice but I it makes me realize that I don't get to do that in my own life.

As I care for them it brings into focus where I am falling short in my own self-care. One reason I can't follow my own advice is the mess in my house from moving and another is that I have been sick and not feeling well enough to do my relaxation exercises. Relaxing at home will hopefully be in my future once we have truly moved in and made the place our own.

Alicia talks about caring for herself as she cared for her mom

When I went down to Puerto Rico to take care of my mother I had the mistaken idea that I would have more time for myself during the time I was there. We had a hospice nurse coming in every morning to bathe her and another woman came in to make the meals and keep the house clean. My main purpose for being there was to keep my mother company and just be with her and not have to do all these other things. I had intended to take care of myself in Puerto Rico even better than at home in New York. I thought that maybe while she was sleeping I could read the books I brought with me or work on a couple of things I needed to do.

When I got there I immediately realized that this was going to be 24/7 and I would really need to make the effort to carve out a little time for myself. I was able to fit it in once she was in bed for the night and had taken all her medicines and was set. I would have a little time to read a book or do a little Yoga or meditation. I only had a little bit of time for myself because I needed to sleep. We would start the whole thing over again the next day at 6 a.m.

Even though we had someone coming in to bathe and dress my mom, I wanted to be a part of that process. I would help with her care instead of leaving or doing my own thing.

I also developed an amazing friendship with the woman who would come in to cook and clean. We still talk after all this time. I used to go with her to the market or dust while she vacuumed a room. As a matter of fact, after my mother died I went back after a few months to visit my dad and I saw that he was living in a pig sty. I asked her back again to cook and clean for him as she had for my mother.

The connections that I made with my new friend and my mother were very special to me. So in a way instead of taking care of myself by reading and getting work done I made a new friend and learned a lot about myself as my mother's Caregiver. I was taking care of myself but in totally unanticipated ways.

Sheri talks about needing to care for herself first

I would reword the question. The more I am able to take care of myself the more I can care for others. If I care for others and don't care for myself I get burnt out. Then my life becomes no good for me and therefore it's no good for others.

It's all about learning self-love. I think that's why we're on this planet to learn self-love. It might take more than one lifetime for some. I learned these lessons with the people I have already cared for and will use this learning when I am called upon to be a Caregiver again in the future.

How does nourishing their needs inform your own need to be nourished?

Alicia talks about maintaining her mother's dignity during her last days

I needed to be with my mom for those last three months because I felt that she needed an advocate by her side. It became my mission in life to support her and I found my role very fulfilling. My need to care for her was as important a consideration for me in my decision to live with her as was my wanting her to experience her power and dignity throughout the dying process. We both benefitted, I could see that.

The way we have Health Care Proxies and Living Wills in the United States... in Puerto Rico they have none of that. There is no legal way to express your end of life wishes. I was concerned that my mother's wishes might be violated and she would be forced to suffer physically but more importantly emotionally. I wanted her to feel her power and be in control of her decisions.

I kept asking the "powers that be" how were we supposed to document my mother's wishes so that we could follow those and not the doctors' wishes? Even asking about it was received as though I didn't care about my mother and just wanted her to be dead. They would also try to gloss over her condition and I would press them to tell me exactly what was happening. They were shocked that I wanted to know all the medical details and that I didn't simply trust the doctor's authority. I wanted my mother to understand the full spectrum of what she was dealing with so she could make educated decisions about her care and her future.

There was one time towards the end that she was home and they wanted to take her back to the hospital for a few days. Everyone started to automatically get ready and call the ambulance. I had to stop everything and ask them when were we going to stop treatments and start following her wishes? She didn't want to go back to the hospital by this point. With my insistence we were able to keep her home and less than a week later she died peacefully in her own bed.

That was my greatest wish for her, to die at home. I didn't trust that her being in a hospital would allow for a very good experience.

She never said anything to me about it, but staying home was something I really wanted for her because I felt it would allow her to have the respect she deserved right to the very end. I felt that allowing her to experience the process of dying at home helped her to keep her dignity intact and that was the main reason I wanted to be with her. Fighting for this helped me to grow into someone who could speak out and not be intimidated by what others would think.

Sheri talks about growing through talking with a friend

I had a friend who would call me because she was going through tough times. Just the process of hearing what I was saying to her helped me because I wanted to practice what I preached. As we aired things out I gained a greater understanding of my own relationships and decisions I had made. It helped me to be stronger and I was able to learn how to receive from her as well so as to keep things balanced.

I generally find it harder to take help than to give it. In this relationship I trust my friend to be there for me. I don't keep track but we can also reverse roles when I need help. We have both benefitted by these conversations by brain storming and supporting each other to grow and solve our problems.

Section E

What caring does to organize our lives and give us meaning

Chapter 23

Caring organizes our life and our priorities

Musings on Mayeroff:
Priorities often change when we start to care for another person. Things that previously mattered in our life can instantly move into the background, allowing issues related to caring to take center stage.[68]

Author's reflections:
Thousands of sons and daughters have unexpectedly quit their jobs and left their homes in haste to live close by to a parent to assume the role of Caregiver. In these cases caring becomes their overriding priority; suddenly, nothing else in their lives matters as much.
In addition, thousands of mothers and fathers have quit their jobs and dropped out of their social circle to care full time for a sick child. Their old life evaporates and is supplanted by a new routine with new priorities.
Other paradigms of Family Caregiving see grandchildren lending a hand to help a frail grandparent; college students will live with and care for grandparents. In the reverse model, a grandparent may care for a grandchild in what has been termed KinCare.
Religious institutions are also instrumental in organizing care within their community as defined by the spirit and values of each denomination.

What priorities have changed in your life based on what you bring to your caring?

Christie talks about her changing priorities as she cared for her husband

I feel like a very different person since I spent the eight years taking care of my husband. I had originally spent three years caring for my grandmother with her cancer but at that time I was unaware of what it meant to be a Caregiver. I just automatically took care of things as a loyal granddaughter would. Those were the values that I had acquired as a young child from my parents and family. She became my priority.

With that experience in my background, I cared for my husband with more awareness of what my role was. I now know that caring is my priority and nothing else in life measures up to the depth of experience I had while caring for him. I was able to live according to my values of caring for others while still being deeply engaged in my life. Caregiving is not a spectator sport and I was happy to have something that challenged me on so many levels. I had a purpose.....

Terry talks about her priorities as she cared for her dad

I value my devotion to my family above all else. When my dad was in hospice I organized my day around my shift - the time I had agreed that I would spend with him. There were no interruptions from work. That was the block of time I kept for the purpose of spending time with my dad. I told everyone that I was unreachable during that time. I had my Blackberry if they needed to send me reports but they knew not to call and knew that I would not be calling them.

At the time the priority wasn't about taking care of myself as much as it was to take care of my parents. I wasn't my own priority anymore, they were. I didn't go on vacation for the 3 years. I didn't socialize as much as I normally would.

Dealing with the stress was a secondary priority for me. I did continue to go to the gym because that was the only way I could keep my strength up and deal with the stress levels. I saw certain things as necessary to remain effective in what I was doing. I value my health and have always worked hard at maintaining it. Going to the gym to work with my trainer was necessary for me to continue to be a Caregiver over the long haul. I would tell my trainer to let me know if I was whining too much but I needed to be there to get the endorphins going and give me a lift.

For me it was the gym. I can imagine that for some people it could be reading a book, cooking or gardening. It doesn't matter. You have to have that space and time in a 24 hour cycle to do something so that you don't totally lose yourself. I also made sure I had my own quiet time to watch TV or anything that would get me away from the sadness or the negativity. I needed time to rejuvenate and think about things I enjoyed thinking about. I had also bought my camera a year before my dad died so I was just starting to get back into photography. This restored my artistic expression and helped me stay on track with my caring.

Since my dad died I've stepped back into my life and savor every minute. I still go to the gym and for my artistic expression I have become immersed in my photography. Even as I still care for my mother this time I have arranged to prioritize myself so I don't get as exhausted as I did while caring for my dad. I've also created better boundaries with my mom and encourage her to take on as much as she can handle for herself.

Musings on Mayeroff:

We tend to become protective of our caring and what is needed to sustain it. The superficialities of life and things we do to merely waste time take a back seat. It now becomes important to shed these things that interfere with the ability to care for someone.[69]

Author's reflections:
Many of us consider that caring is what gives us our purpose in life. Caring for a family member will often take precedence over other responsibilities. Not even the responsibilities of our employment can compare to our need to make sure our family members and friends are well cared for.

Businesses have been made to understand the toll Caregiving can take on one's job performance. Many of them have started to offer services to relieve the burdens that Caregivers face. Flex time, working from home and offering onsite emotional support are an example of some of the programs that have been incorporated into the work place to relieve Caregiver stress.

When a family member falls ill, Caregivers try to limit their outside responsibilities in order to provide adequate care for this person they are caring for. At its most demanding, Caregiving can make everyday responsibilities seem superfluous. At the same time, meeting those everyday demands that cannot be ignored can leave the Caregiver conflicted and feeling as if they were neglecting the person they are caring for. Just a trip to the grocery store can cause the Caregiver extra worry and guilt for leaving.

What do you do when situations and people interfere with your ability to care?

Christie talks about fitting her schedule around caring for her grandmother

During the time that I was taking care of my grandmother, while she was in the hospital, I was also in massage school and working. I would visit her in the evening after work and sometimes wouldn't get there until 10 p.m.

When my schedule interfered with my ability to care for my grandmother, I just worked around it and extended my day. The nurses knew me and let me come in after the official visiting hours were over. I would get updates on her condition and when she needed 24 hour nursing care I arranged for that. It was a very stressful time but I didn't let my work or school schedule stop me from helping as much as I could.

At one point during this time I started feeling that something was wrong with my health. My doctor had me wear a heart monitor for a week. He told me that my heart would race sometimes due to the stress. Since I was an athlete I was still in a safe zone but it showed me how my health was being damaged by the situation. It also taught me that in order to continue to care for my grandmother I would have to find ways to relax or manage the stress better. I had always valued my health but I now saw the Caregiving had taken over as my priority and my health suffered.

Terry talks about getting good medical care for her dad

I got really pissed when others got in the way of my being able to properly care for my dad. The office people were telling me that he wasn't scheduled for a PET scan for another 3 months. His doctor needed to find out right now how much the cancer had progressed so he could decide what treatment would be best. We couldn't wait for their rigid schedule of testing to kick in.

I remember screaming at them on the cellphone in the middle of Macy's in the dishware department. "My father has lung cancer. I don't care about your rules, these rules need to be broken. This is my father's life you are talking about here. We aren't asking for these tests for the fun of it!"

My passion and anger increased to the 'nth degree when it had to do with something so critical and then someone I am dealing with decides to tell me no. There are no exceptions. My priority was to protect my dad. This comes out of how close my family is and how much we value each other. Nothing will get in the way of our ability to care.

Musings on Mayeroff:
A caring person tends to gravitate towards other caring people. Because they share similar experiences they can encourage and support each other in their caring.[70]

Author's reflections:
Just as runners join running clubs and set times to run together, and just as musicians plan rehearsals or go out to hear music together, Caregivers tend to find others in their same situation. It's not as easy of course. There aren't many drop-in centers for Caregivers and there isn't a certain way of dressing that would help them pick each other out in the grocery store.

When they do find each other they immediately see that they share many ethical concerns, along with experiences and emotions. They can recognize similar accommodations that they have had to make in their lives and don't question each other's overriding commitment to their caring as a non-Caregiver might.

Have you met other Caregivers and shared commonalities with them?

Christie talks about finding other husbands and wives who had cared for their spouses

Once my husband was moved to a nursing home for the last year and a half of his life I was able to get out more and explore our town. We had been living there for seven years, but I was kept home with my Caregiving for much of that time. He and I would venture into town for music and jam sessions but I was always kept busy with him and wasn't making new friends.

Just before he was placed in the nursing home, I met my new friend Barb. From her I was able to find out about community groups to join and places to meet new people. She sponsored me and I joined Rotary which immediately opened up my world, since ours is a large club of local business owners and community leaders. I did immediately find other members whose spouses had already died. They would tell me their stories of sadness and how they picked up and kept going.

Two of the Rotary women were still taking care of their husbands who had had strokes or other health issues. We bonded and eventually we each lost our husband. We supported each other with a deep knowing that we had all been through a similar experience, the loss of a loved one, pride that we had cared for them and the rebuilding of our lives that followed. We had made similar decisions to devote ourselves to our caring based on our shared view of what was important and what brought meaning to us in our lives.

Terry talks about finding friends in similar situations

A lot of my friends have been through difficult situations like mine. I feel much more at ease talking to people who have been through similar Caregiving experiences. They understand the flow of emotions and the various decisions that have to be made. We share beliefs and values about our need to care and our responsibilities to do it well. People who haven't been through it can't understand how you can give so much of yourself to another. They especially don't see what you get back.

Are you able to support other Caregivers when you meet them?

Christie talks about speaking with recent widows

Through my volunteer work at the hospital I often come in contact with wives who are caring for critically ill husbands. Even when they have no idea of my history, I have a feeling that there is a deep sense of understanding that I can communicate just by listening to their struggles.

My guess is that if you asked most people they would tell you that their biggest fear would be to lose their spouse or their child. By volunteering I get to support parents, wives and husbands who are going through this worst thing that they have ever imagined.

Terry talks about her friends who were Caregivers

It was important to have people around who I could call and talk to when things got tough. They were travelling a similar path and I supported them when they were crashing. Someone like this would know instantly what I was going through and provided a place for me to vent. It was also important that they were outside my family. I felt freer with them.

Sometimes my Caregiver friend and I would go out to dinner and end up just holding each other's hands and crying. The other people in the restaurant probably thought we were breaking up or something.

Musings on Mayeroff:
When we organize our lives around caring we may need to give up certain other aspects of our life. This might be experienced as a sub-

mission to a higher goal. Since this deprivation is associated with the goal of caring it resembles other commitments like our hobbies or any sports we may be involved with.

Athletes subject themselves to their training regimes and artists spend many hours devoted to their work. They might lose an active social life but there is little focus on what they are losing. Their priority is more on what is being gained.

Doubts and second guessing can cripple the life of someone who has not found something or someone to be devoted to. The certainty of what is required for sports or art or Caregiving is both freeing and builds confidence due to the clarity of what is required to accomplish each. [71]

Author's reflections:
When a Caregiver starts on their journey of caring there are many sacrifices to be made. It's a funny thing, however, that many Caregivers do not experience these sacrifices resentfully or as a deprivation. It is often described as feeling like "it comes with the territory."

There is no training to become a Family Caregiver and Caregivers aren't warned ahead of time about what will be expected of them. Many of them are able to devote vast amounts of their time and energy without hesitation. Having found a purpose in their life can energize Caregivers beyond any expectation they'd had of themselves or others had had of them.

How do you experience the fact that, as a Caregiver, there are things in your life that you have had to give up?

Christie talks about what she had to give up to care for her husband

At first I didn't have to give up much because my husband was young and healthy and more willing than ever to do things together. My life became richer for many years. As I looked for things that he would like to do we got to take the time to visit museums, see movies, visit with friends and get out into nature.

This went on for many years until the Alzheimer's started to catch up with him. He became weaker, more disoriented and less motivated. That was hard for me because it was more difficult for me to still do the things I loved. I remember taking him snow shoeing and having to listen to him complaining the whole time. The silence of the snow covered world was shattered but at least we were out of the house. These were the things I had to gradually give up.

Money was a big issue throughout my caring for him. I ultimately had to give up our financial security. At first it was a matter of the lack of his income as he was no longer able to work with computers or eventually teach music. He had Social Security but that was a fraction of what he used to earn. I started to have to make up the difference. Luckily I had just graduated from acupuncture school and was bringing in good money for several years. He eventually had to come with me to the office and that meant that I could only work a day and a half a week. This is when our finances really started to suffer. Since we had the house I had a home equity line of credit and just before he died I had maxed out on that. Five years after his passing I am slowly regaining my financial stability. I still have a huge loan to pay back but I am clear about my future and goals. In the meanwhile I carefully budget and now have support from my new boyfriend when I need it.

Terry talks about what she had to give up as she took care of her dad

I gave up my vacations during the time I cared for my dad. At the time I didn't resent it but now I wish I had gone. I can see more clearly that it would have helped me emotionally. I used to feel guilty going on a business trip for a week. I worried that something might happen to my dad or that the family would need me for something. Obviously by the time he was in hospice I wasn't going anywhere, but before that I could have done something for myself. Since there was me, my sister, brother and mom I could have gone away.

Everyone else except me and my mom had ways to disconnect from the situation. For someone who is a solo Caregiver they would have a different decision to make and my mom certainly wouldn't have felt comfortable leaving my dad.

In terms of my social life and the friends I didn't see for a couple of years, some I have re-connected with and others I haven't. I still haven't resumed the social life I had before. It's slowly rebuilding itself but it takes time. I'm also probably still grieving and honestly I'm depressed when I get home at night. I turn on the TV and I don't really want to talk to anybody. I don't want to do anything. I want to be left alone.

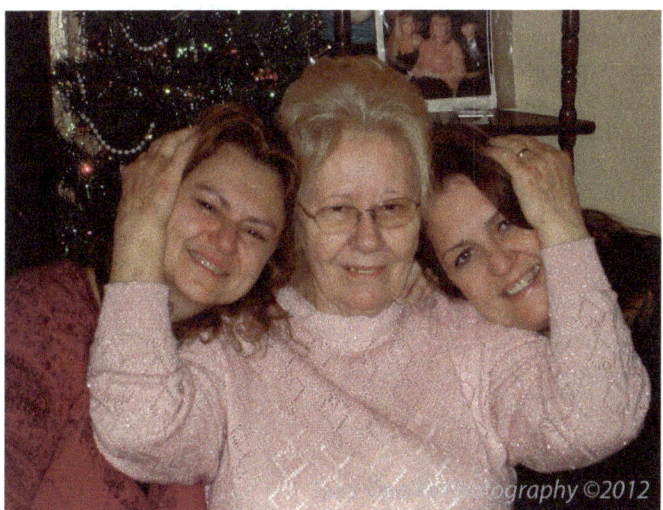

Terry and her mom and sister

Have the changes you have had to make as a Caregiver had a positive outcome?

Christie talks about the positive outcomes of caring for her husband

Most likely once my husband was placed in the nursing home I would have withdrawn from business and work if I had had the money available to take some time off. Instead, partly due to my financial situation, I had to get out there and meet new people. This had a positive effect on me because all of this required a certain amount of confidence and outgoingness.

When I think back to even five years ago, I considered myself shy with new people and a bit of a recluse. All that changed after my husband died. I started meeting more people and being exposed to new ideas. All of that requires me to be outgoing and confident.

Terry talks about having better boundaries while caring for her mother as a positive outcome

I realize how important it is to separate and I can go on vacations now. I now have the comfort to be able to take time away when I need it. I'm not held back by thinking that now my mother needs me and I shouldn't leave. I explain to her that we'll take care of things when I get back and that I need to leave. I don't feel that I have to drop everything about me to do for her. I sometimes feel the guilt but I also feel that she is too attached and dependent on me and there needs to be a line that is drawn between us. I need to have my own life and start dating. I put that aside for 3 years after all!

I enjoy doing for my mom. I even like to travel with her. We went to Florida to see my elderly aunt. At first she didn't want to go but I convinced her that this might be their last chance to see each other. I want to take her to England next year. But that being said I also want to have time to be free from her. I talk to her every day on the phone. If a few days pass she calls me and is all worried. My friends hear that we speak every day and they are surprised since they might talk to their moms once a week or less. I've always talked to my mom every day but sometimes I need a break. I didn't feel this way when I was caring for my dad so I think this is a positive change in me.

Chapter 24

The music of caring: themes, harmony and flow

Musings on Mayeroff:
When our caring is all-embracing, it provides us a focal point with certain themes around which our day-to-day life revolves as we move into a deeply flowing harmony with the world.72 (p. 54)

Author's reflections:
Since harmony is the blending of compatible vibrations and we generally think of it in the context of music, musical harmony becomes an excellent metaphor for caring.

Flow is the movement forward. In music this flow can be smooth, choppy, swinging, rigid or formal. In Caregiving, depending on the day, there is also a flow. Tasks that need doing, meals that need preparing, medicines that need dispensing, doctors that need to be visited and comfort that needs tending to. When all goes according to plan there is a smooth flow. When the person being cared for is having a bad day the flow may become choppy. When the Caregiver is having a bad day and the flow is obstructed hopelessness and overwhelm can enter and take over the flow and everything falls apart.

Themes are also useful to look at through the lens of Caregiving. Themes are the "thoughts" in music. Themes group musical passages together into recognizable melodic units. Caregiving also carries themes and repeated patterns that are recognizable. Hyper-vigilance with nearly constant concern might be one of these themes that many Caregivers experience.

When musical notes are random--when the notes don't reach for harmony and have no direction or flow--except for extreme modernists, we wouldn't call it music but cacophony, which is the random grouping of sounds or notes. We would most likely put our hands over our ears if an ambulance drove by with its siren screeching and horns honking, disturbed by the cacophony. The EMS team in this example is trying to get our attention, but because of the anarchy of their sound, they could not connect with us in any but the most fleeting and disagreeable way, making achieving a harmonious communication impossible.

In Caregiving it's important for us to feel comfortable, in harmony essentially, with our responsibilities. When families clash or friends quarrel there is, to borrow from the literal meaning of the word, discord; each person becomes isolated leaving the field ripe for burnout and depression. On the other hand, when those involved in a patient's care are "in tune" with each other, dissonance falls away and the person being cared for, the central theme of the caring endeavor, is comforted.

For many Caregivers, those who were formerly involved in caring too, the experience often doesn't feel like a sacrifice or an arduous task. Often they will describe the sense of purpose they feel or once felt as a Caregiver and, in day-to-day terms, the comfort that knowing exactly what is expected of them brings them. These Caregivers have found the music in their Caregiving. They have experienced the positive satisfaction between the harmony, flow and themes in their own life as Caregivers which erases negativity, self-doubt and yearning for something more.

Are there central themes in your life that determine how you live? Give some examples.

Claudine talks about her own life and its themes

Yes I have two themes. The first one is illness and my role as a Caregiver. I had taken care of my mother who had diabetes when I was younger. Then I left Canada, thinking I could leave illness behind. I married a young healthy man. Now he has the same disease as my mother and I am starting all over again. I have to deal with his diabetes on a daily basis. His illness is always there and I am always monitoring his foods, exercise and variations in his health due to his changing blood sugar levels. Because of my mother I am familiar with these daily themes of Caregiving.

My daughter also has health issues that I have become involved with. In her case since no one can figure out what is wrong with her the flow of my care for her is choppy and intermittent. Her blood work always has abnormal readings but they can't pin down what is going on. Since I am her mother she only comes to me when she is falling apart and afraid of what she might finally learn about her health. Worry is a constant theme for me.

Abandonment is the other theme in my life. My mother was a neglected child and now my husband is also a neglected child. And even I was neglected in a different way. My mother, being hyper-vigilant, ironically couldn't trust herself or a nanny to care for me so she sent me away to a boarding school where I felt very un-cared for and abandoned by my family. I would never want to do that to someone I love so I have become highly committed to my caring for my husband and my daughter and even for myself. This has clearly been a unifying theme for me even when it is a struggle. The challenges give me purpose and the fact that I can offer this level of caring to the two people I love the most gives me great satisfaction.

Debbie talks about the themes that run through her life

My themes come from my spiritual work. My Yoga teacher who is also a counselor as a Social Worker would connect me to what we were learning in class as to how I could apply it to what I was experiencing with my Caregiving for my mom. I depended heavily on our sessions, so much so that I often remind myself that I got through my Caregiving situation with both the support of my Yoga practice and that of my teacher when I needed more clarity.

I always had the feeling I was doing the right thing in my caring even though on the surface it may have seemed more random. Looking back I never felt like I had to directly take care of my mom. I was really caring more directly for my sister who was reaching the end of her rope and calling to the rest of the family for help.

One of the themes that is important in Yoga is to do no harm. There was a trailer on the land behind my mother's house. All of it was going into foreclosure because my mother, the owner, wasn't paying her bills. She had rented the trailer to a cousin. He told us that she had said she would sell him the house and property. By now she no longer had the right to sell the house or the trailer because technically the bank owned it. Before I called him about it I took a deep breath and remembered that I would do no harm to myself by getting angry. In my head I was saying the mantra of "do no harm". He escalated and I de-escalated. In short order he calmed down. It helped to remember that he was angry at the situation and not at me personally. I also learned that from my Yoga training. It was very satisfying for me to know that my behavior could have such a positive effect on our interaction.

It was harder to follow my spiritual practices when dealing directly with my mom. She could push my buttons. I did the best I could and I did also prepare myself to be calm before I spoke to her on the phone. I would remind my sister to do the same thing before speaking with her. Regardless of our good intentions it is harder when it is your mother. That's where my Yoga teacher was such a help. I was finally able to open my heart and be more accepting of my mother's idiosyncrasies.

How does your caring fit into the themes in your life?

Claudine talks about forming a new caring family with her neighbors

Out of the theme of having experienced abandonment I learned how to create a new type of family for my daughter. I never wanted her to feel isolated or abandoned the way my husband and I had. As my husband and I care for our daughter we have created a new type of family out of the friends and neighbors we love. Since I'm isolated from my biological family because I moved away from Canada and my husband's family abandoned him for emotional reasons, we have had to raise our daughter without any support from our families.

We created a new form of family by blending our family with those of our neighbors and friends. Our next door neighbors would take our daughter in the mornings and after school we would have their kids over on the weekend when their mom was working. Our daughter regarded them as her sisters. Since she was able to experience these close bonds she didn't ever have to feel emotionally abandoned the way her father and I have.

As a teen our daughter started babysitting two kids whose parents both worked long hours. My husband and I were sensitive to their needs and basically helped raise those two kids. They still come over all the time when they see that our daughter is visiting. The older kid considers our daughter to be her big sister. The younger one still stops to say hello to us when she is riding her bike with her friends. There is a real harmony in our community as we all work to care for each other and build broader definitions of what it means to be a family and give our daughter a form of connection that we didn't have.

Debbie talks about finding harmony in caring for her mother

When it came to the theme of acceptance I had to learn to accept that my mother wouldn't always tell me the truth. This was her quirk. It helped to talk to my aunt and realize that my mother had had these issues from childhood. It wasn't something new or something she only would do with me. I just had to accept that she would keep doing this.

It was hard as a child to accept that she wouldn't always tell the truth. We depended on her for truth and she couldn't provide that. I wanted her to be honest with me and when she wasn't I was always disappointed.

As an adult I worked on being able to accept this about her but it was very difficult. Instead of harmony there was confusion and doubt about what she would tell us. As I grew more accepting through my work with my Yoga teacher and my Yoga practice I could see that this was just a symptom. It was a behavior that only represented a small part of who she was and we were finally able to blend together in a more loving way. It wasn't perfect but it was improving. If I had had more time with my mom I think we were headed towards a more harmonious relationship.

Musings on Mayeroff:
Our personal experience with caring brings us into harmony with the rest of the world.[73]

Author's reflections:
Even though many Caregivers are isolated in their day to day caring and many are even ruggedly individualistic and reluctant to ask for help no Caregiver is ever completely alone. There is a harmony and a flow that connect Caregivers to their communities, like it or not.

Caregiving is the job of an activist. They are the ones to create a harmony with their surroundings. Many Caregivers change from being relatively passive about life to becoming the championing advocate for the person they are caring for. It's the "mama bear" syndrome. Mother bears in the wild will maul anyone that even comes near their cubs. Caregivers have been known to scream in hospital corridors, burst into doctors' offices unannounced and make hundreds of calls to unresponsive insurance companies on behalf of the person they are caring for.

They have been able to nurture an assertiveness they didn't know they had and can now ask questions, disagree with authority figures and get the best outcomes for those they are providing care to. They are creating a smooth flow and a blended harmony with those they come in contact with. It's not easy and it often fails but the Caregiver bravely goes on to try another day.

As a Caregiver's commitment to a loved one or family comes to an end, increasingly more of them will become involved in helping those outside their own family. When they find each other and join forces, Caregivers can be a vocal group seeking to fulfill patients' needs with former Caregivers there to support them. Caregiver advocacy groups are looking for ways to create harmony between what is needed and what is being offered by the community. Caregivers experienced lack of support and animosity in the face of their daunting task and know firsthand how frequently patients are deprived of necessary services; and from being on the front lines they also know firsthand what would improve an inefficient and bureaucratic system of service supply. This movement is in its infancy but with an exponentially growing need it is certain to expand quickly.

Has being a Caregiver made you more proactive in your commitments?

Claudine talks about becoming more active in finding a better teaching position

Because I cared for my parents I experienced how that situation energized me and how much I grew as a person during that time. In contrast at my former teaching job I was passive for a long while hoping that I could advance within the school but they never picked me to move up. I found that it was becoming more and more difficult to have the energy to care for my work and my students. There was no harmony or flow between myself and the school administration. I wasn't growing and it was interfering with my creativity and what I could hope to accomplish. I felt like I was swimming in dead waters or even against a current at certain times. There was not a flow that was carrying me along.

So recently I decided to change things. I became more active about finally leaving my job after five years of this discontent with the status quo. It meant returning to promoting my skills and the things I know about education and the system. It was interesting that by becoming more active I was out in the world looking for opportunities but these two new jobs actually sought me out in the end. I felt a harmony between my talents and what others were looking for. I can say that in my new job I'm more energized, there is a flow and as a result I can give more of myself to my students. I can feel the circumstances are now more harmonious and I feel appreciated for what I can give to others. I can feel myself starting to grow as a person again which is very rewarding to me.

Debbie talks about actively caring for her son

I would say I'm more active in my commitments to my family since caring for my mother. My son would probably say I'm too active. He's been telling me when I need to back off. I may have gone a bit overboard. Sometimes when I strive for harmony and flow with my son his needs aren't being met and I have to change my course. I see that now. I'm getting better at listening to his needs and taking my direction from him so there is more harmony in our interactions.

Things have improved recently and my son is creating a non-profit to help people and I'm only supporting him when he asks me to. I've talked to my sister about it and she thinks it is good to let your kids succeed on their own or even fail once in a while. That's how they learn. There is definitely more peace in our ability to work together on his project.

I see now that when my sisters and I look at our kids we can be proud that they had a more secure upbringing and can relax more in their lives then we were able to. There is more harmony and flow to how we have raised them even though we had to learn an entirely new way of being parents from how our parents raised us.

Do you feel connected now in a more harmonious way to the world and to other Caregivers because of your Caregiving experience?

Claudine talks about being connected to others who care

I do feel connected to others who care. I also look for how to create harmony in the relationships I have. It seems easier to do this with others who are caring and thoughtful. I try to surround myself with people who are generous and caring now. That may be because of an understanding I acquired as I cared for my parents and now caring for my husband and daughter with their health issues. Caregivers are a great bunch of people and I believe that they understand more about the truths of life. I find it easier to be around them these days because the themes that direct our lives are similar.

My husband and daughter are very caring and I enjoy being with them. Harmony in my family is important to me. I also see how they, each of them, behaves outside of our home and am very proud of them. When my husband is at work in his construction job, many of his co-workers come to him with their problems. He gives them emotional and sometimes financial support. My daughter is also very caring with her friends. I see that. There is a real flow in each of their lives as they energize those around them.

Caring has been an ever present theme in my life. Many of the women at the school that I left were battling breast cancer, so they needed my care. They would also need my support when their parents were either dying or needing to be placed in facilities. They seemed to feel that they could talk to me about all of it because I had been in their shoes. This is a gift I have and can offer to others. I can see how to bring groups like these teachers together into more harmonious relationships.

Debbie talks about being attracted to other Caregivers

Yes, I'm involved with Caregivers right in my own family. It seems to be a theme for all of us. My younger sister is a nurse practitioner. The older one is still dealing with at risk teens. It seems to be my life's work to connect with caring people like my Yoga teacher. That's who I hang out with, that's who I'm attracted to.

Now all I want is to create harmony in the situations I am in with the people who want the same things. This wasn't always true when I was younger but I've grown into this connection since supporting and caring for my mother and sister. I get it now. As I look for ways to give back and volunteer I have chosen Caregivers as the group I would like to support most. I have joined an organization that helps connect Family Caregivers to support and resources. I can see as a former dancer the effect that I have in creating a sort of musical flow and harmony out of the challenges that Caregivers experience.

Chapter 25

The feeling of being "in place" or "at home" in our world

Musings on Mayeroff:
Experiencing the feeling of being "in place" is a dynamic process with which we continually interact. The clarity of our own purpose that we get when we respond to the other person's need to grow reflects the "in place" feeling we get from this interaction.[74]

Author's reflections:
When we move to a new home we try to make it feel comfortable and "homey". This is how we achieve a sense of well-being in our physical world. We may hang familiar and favorite artwork on the walls or find just the right spot for our favorite chair.

On the emotional front, the combination of three elements, comfort, caring and challenge gives us a feeling of being "at home" within ourselves and a sense of equilibrium: we feel comforted by our routines, we use our caring to establish a feeling of purpose, and we need challenges in our life and work in order to feel personal satisfaction.

Often the ability to have all three in our lives, our feeling of comfort, a relationship that causes us to care deeply and lifelong learning with its challenges, isn't possible. When we focus on one of these three elements to the exclusion of the other two we risk feeling unsettled. Sometimes life gets boring and repetitive because we are not challenging ourselves by deepening our life's experience. Or, we maybe didn't appreciate the importance that caring for others holds as one of the ways to find peace and meaning in our lives. At other times life is full of new horizons and challenges but we forget to step back and take some down time to comfort and center ourselves, reflect, and plan the best ways for meeting those challenges.

When one of these three elements is missing, we may feel awkward, "out of place" emotionally, or feel generally disconnected, like a "stranger in a strange land". One may become restless over time, often with impulse to escape. This can happen in our jobs or in our relationships. We start wandering away from our original purpose looking for something to restore our feeling of comfort or give us some satisfaction. We surround ourselves with possessions to comfort us but they don't help us to find our meaning and purpose in the world. This is a feeling that needs to be cultivated through our engagement in a well-integrated life that includes caring, comfort, challenge, openness to learning, and time to reflect.[75]

The quickest and truest way to feel "in place" with ourselves is to connect to the process of deeply caring for another. As we experience the satisfaction of watching another person thrive thanks to our attentiveness, we also boost our self-gratification. We know our path is the right one because we see the results of our caring and experience our own growth in the challenge of the process.

Do you feel comfortable with your place in the world?

Christie talks about Caregiving as a central theme

Yes, it has taken a lifetime to feel this way. I have a certainty now about what my life is about. It grew directly out of my experiences as a Caregiver for my grandmother and husband and probably even started earlier as the oldest sister of four siblings.

I remember looking into all my challenges as an athlete or a musician to find a central theme but nothing was all inclusive for me. I still felt restless and needed to search further.

Only after having the time for reflecting on my many years spent as a Caregiver did I realize this very Caregiving had pulled everything together. My past connected to my future and the entire process of Caregiving was challenging and creative, which satisfied my soul. I now make time in my life for reflection, sharing, challenges and caring for others. It's perfect!

Julie talks about preferring to feel comfortable

I usually feel comfortable with my place in the world unless I'm feeling irritable or scared and then I don't. I still find myself being a Caregiver for my friends who are experiencing serious health issues. I am still on an emotional roller coaster as they deal with heart attacks and kidney failure rather than head colds and the flu like when we were all younger. I don't especially like these challenges.

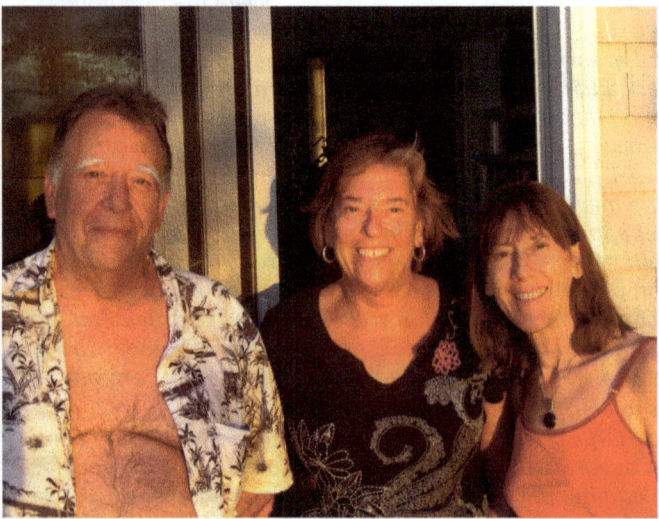

Julie (rt.) with her sister and brother.

My problem with all this is thinking that my place in the world should include these challenges but not always feeling comfortable with them. I haven't yet embraced the idea of challenge or seen the benefits of this level and intensity of Caregiving. I fall into feeling that I should be comfortable all the time even when I'm afraid and not feeling "in place". I'm not there yet.

Author's reflections:
There is a question that every child is prompted to answer at least a hundred times and that's "What do you want to be when you grow up?" Some kids know immediately how to answer that question. They pick someone they have seen: a teacher at school, a nurse in a clinic, a parent who is a police officer, a favorite aunt who is a scientist, and this helps them choose a career path. Sometimes they figure out that the arts are calling to them and they pick up a musical instrument or a paintbrush, a pen for writing or a glittery costume for dance.

And then there are those who must search hard for their unique place. They don't want to be boxed into an early decision that doesn't fit or can't be altered. These are the restless spirits among us. They need time to find their place in the world.

Fast forward to when the time comes to take on the role of Caregiver with its potential for personal satisfaction and certainty. Instead of being in a position to embrace the role of Caregiver many of us find ourselves in distant locations feeling guilty and untethered to any significant meaning in our lives. Working long hours, paying our bills and having busy social lives take the place of feeling connected to someone who really needs us.

Feeling that we have found our place in the world has very little to do with what others want for us. When we are called on to be Caregivers for our parents, or grandparents, aunts or uncles, husbands or wives we are being asked to make many decisions about our futures and theirs.

This is something that only we can figure out for ourselves. We have to make all the small and large choices about how we want to live. We need to feel that these choices are a good fit for us. Finding our place in the world is a dynamic process. Others cannot do this work for us. When parents or others push too hard for us to be there for them our ability to explore our choices gets stunted. Listening to our inner feelings and knowing our strengths guide us towards being truly "at home" with ourselves.

Many of the adult children who are able to move back and can make that decision to be the primary Caregiver for their parents, other relatives or even childhood friends experience the satisfaction that comes from Caregiving. The public looks at what they may have given up, a good job, a nice car but what outsiders don't see is what the experience of Caregiving can bring. There is often a feeling of everything being right or "in place" that starts to grow as the Caregiver finds comfort in the challenges and routines that become their life.

Musings on Mayeroff:
Fulfilling interactions with other caring people allow us to bond in ways that help us to feel "at home" with others and to grasp what it means to be "in place" in our communities.[76]

Author's reflections:
We have spoken about the inner feeling of being "in place" but feeling "in place" can also relate to our outside relationships; positive community relationships contrast the other reality of impersonal communities isolated by a materialism symbolized by the gated, fortress-like homes that have proliferated of late. But caring for others and growing strong communities with resources to fall back on when needed is a much stronger approach to a true sense of comfort, peace and security for the entire group.

How have others helped you find that "in place" feeling?

Christie talks about her neighbors

When my husband and I first moved upstate and bought a house we were welcomed by our neighbors on either side of our new home. One family welcomed us as part of their extended family. We shared many a story over the backyard fence in addition to helping them locate their many rescue dogs or cats who had wandered off their property. When my husband took a turn for the worse and started hallucinating with his Alzheimer's they came over and cared for him until I got back home. They were very compassionate and helped us to feel very settled in our new home.

On the other side of our house there was a wonderful Irish fellow who would share meals with us and as my husband's health declined he would do some of the heavy lifting in our garden or helped when it was time to move heavy furniture. He was a wonderful soul and also gave us a sense that we "belonged" in our new home and community.

Our new home was located in a larger Colony that had an eighty year history of political activity and cultural events. Through the Colony we learned about how neighbors were coming together to keep the communal lake healthy. Through the annual events we were able to play music with our neighbors, share meals at the beach and enjoy the story-telling festival. In order to stay connected I would bring my husband to the monthly board of director meetings and we got to hear about the problems, challenges and successes of the Colony. We definitely had the feeling that we belonged to something larger in our community.

Julie talks about feeling comfortable with others

I belong to a group of women who are acupuncturists. We are a caring group and have chosen to socialize with each other. We often combine work and pleasure, like taking trips to seminars and then sharing rooms and social time in the evenings.

I always feel welcomed in my friends' houses. I don't go to places where I don't feel comfortable. I'm not a sociable being at this point.

I feel welcomed into my clients' lives as an acupuncturist and my relationship with them is based on that. I also felt comfortable and welcomed as a teacher at the acupuncture school by the students.

Musings on Mayeroff:
Everyone is capable of being "in place" through caring.[77]

Author's reflections:
Once a Caregiver gets the hang of what true caring is, recognizing it as mutual support and good will and, at times, flourishing, it can become the central axis of their life.

Mayeroff mentions the additional caring for our work, our sports, our art, our spirituality, science or anything that fulfills us. All of these carings have the potential to give us a feeling of being "in place" with ourselves, but in my mind nothing matches the caring that we offer each other, especially when someone is vulnerable, as in Caregiving. There is the potential for a deep inner sense of well-being that develops from a Caregiving relationship.

Does your caring for others give you a feeling of well-being and purpose?

Christie talks about finding purpose in caring for her husband

When I took care of my husband when he started showing signs of dementia there wasn't a day that went by where I resented my role. Of course there were plenty of difficult days but the overall sense was that I had a purpose. He needed me and I could be there for him. This clarity of purpose made my decision to take on this role way more simple than anything else I've ever taken on. It certainly contributed to an over-all sense of well-being for me.

I hear Caregivers saying they didn't have a choice and at the time I felt the same way. Years later I understand that we all have the choice. We willing Caregivers have accepted our roles and the lack of our resistance makes this decision feel almost effortless. It is clear to most that Caregiving isn't for everyone and others make different choices.

My Caregiver role was comfortable for me as long as my husband and I were in our little cocoon of a life. When I took him out it was more complicated and a challenge to navigate social events. I still felt that I was clear about my role and if it meant translating what he had just said or making sure he didn't get lost it was all in a day's work. It made me happy and gave me a sense of meaning and purpose to be able to offer my husband a full life, despite his Alzheimer's.

Julie talks about finding purpose in caring for her mother and friends

Caring comes into my life in a variety of ways. I usually accept my role as Caregiver when I feel that I am the one looking to see how I can help and offering what I feel able to give.

When she was alive and being treated for her cancer I was frequently going to Rhode Island and taking my mother to her transfusions. I definitely felt a sense of purpose and really enjoyed it. I also enjoy caring for my acupuncture clients because I feel like I am really helping them. I've also enjoyed helping my friends both emotionally and with concrete assistance. I've helped a certain friend a lot during her divorce and relocation. When another friend's husband was sick I felt that it was important for me to support her in the way that I could. That's a big part of how I define myself and who I am. I show up to help when I am needed by my close friends, like when my first boyfriend got sick recently.

It's important and I do feel very good about caring for others. It can even happen out of the blue. I ran into a teacher from school and she was having an awful day and needed to get to three different places. I happened to be there with my car and so I could help her and it was a total lift for me. Even years ago when I was a waitress I wanted people to really enjoy their dinner and I wanted to be a part of that.

And with massage I wanted it to be very special for people. One of my clients had a rough experience at her first massage in a Korean spa. When I did acupuncture near her feet she would break out in a sweat of anxiety. I was able to massage her feet gently so that she could start to enjoy massage and also be less anxious about her acupuncture sessions. To know that I had given her this positive experience with massage was really fun for me.

I feel entirely differently when someone is demanding or trying to manipulate me. My friend who has a mental illness has been one of my best teachers. When she asks for money, even though she has a full time job, and I don't really know if she has money for food, I refuse to give it unless it's a loan. I've learned that I love to give and care but it has to be more on my terms and boundaries are important.

Musings on Mayeroff:
When our caring allows us to engage our strengths and talents, it allows us to feel "in place".[78]

Author's reflections:
In Positive Psychology the various techniques used to promote happiness and fulfillment are studied. Positive Psychology doesn't merely slap positive thoughts over difficulties. Researchers in the field have shown that by changing our perspective, engaging fully in life, and above all using our strengths and talents fully, things like the ability to listen, have empathy or be patient, we can feel proud of our endeavors, more fulfilled and "at home" with ourselves.

Which strengths are you using in your caring?

Christie talks about the strengths she used while caring for her husband

I put to use many of my strengths during the eight years that I cared for my husband but I don't think I could have named them at the time. Upon looking back over the years I can see that caring for someone with Alzheimer's requires an almost super human amount of imagination and flexibility of thought. When people ask me about how I handled certain behaviors it almost always comes down to my ability to change my idea of what was "normal". Alzheimer's brings with it a "new normal" for the person going through it and the Caregiver has to go with the flow if there is to be any peace at all. My strength was my flexibility of thought.

Thankfully my years and years of being a jazz musician and knowing how to improvise came in handy when caring for my husband. There was never a limit to what I would do to try to keep things fun and flexible. I would make up silly plays and have the two of us act out roles. I would find other ways to re-direct his concerns when he got fixated on things.

Because I have always been an athlete and planning and strategy are important to my training and competing I was able to apply this ability to strategize to being a Caregiver. Problems would present themselves and eventually after trial and error I would find a solution. I had the ability to stay with a temporary failure and keep working to eventually find a solution that would work. Sometimes it would take over a month to get it right. Athletes are used to looking at the long term to plan and be able to accomplish their goals. Quick fixes rarely work in the world of sports. This talent for planning felt familiar to me and also helped me time and again in my Caregiving.

Now that my Caregiving is in the past I am surprised at the level of confidence I have when I enter new situations. I have felt comfortable speaking with anyone from the president of a hospital to a politician or a nationally known figure. I seem to know myself and my qualities and can clearly see how different this clarity is from my pre-Caregiving days.

Julie talks about the strengths she uses in her caring

I'm perceptive and have a good sense of what is going on with another person. I have good hands for healing. I'm great at giving advice and I love doing it. I was a really good teacher. I can be funny and make people laugh. I used humor a lot when I was a teacher because I could see the students panicking and I remembered what it was like to be in their shoes and so frightened.

I also teach my clients about their health and the concepts that Chinese Medicine offers. For the clients who want to know more I really enjoy my teaching role. I am also trustworthy and can feel compassion. If someone is crying I'll cry with them. There is no better purpose to have in life as far as I'm concerned. Sharing myself with others is all I really need to do to feel a comfort with myself and realize what is most important to me.

Chapter 26
Significant others

Musings on Mayeroff:
Our relationships with our significant others evolve until they become the pivotal center around which our life revolves.[79]

Author's reflections:
When we look back over our lives we start to recognize the importance of the relationships that have guided us. Often we tell our story based on the important people and relationships in our lives. These important people don't have to be our spouse or lover. The word significant in this Caregiving context reflects our priorities.

A significant other can be the frail mother that the son is focused on caring for or the child who their parents focus on and become advocates for acquire the extra accommodations they need at school.

As we get older we notice ourselves describing events as they relate to before or after a significant someone's death or marriage or the birth of a child. In this indirect way we can already start to absorb how our lives revolve around these relationships we consider the pillars of our journey.

Does someone that you care for serve as the central focus of your life?

Barbara talks about her life as it revolves around her two children

Now that my husband is gone my life totally revolves around my kids. It's too much really. My ego is completely lost inside of their accomplishments and their failures. I feel that everything they do is a direct reflection on me. I haven't been able to separate myself from their lives, and in my opinion this is totally wrong. I hope I live long enough for them to outgrow the damage I've done.

Olivia speaks of caring for her significant others: her middle brother and her mother

During my life I have cared for many people and at each juncture when they required increased care they sequentially became my significant other. My middle brother was a veteran and for three years he lived with me or on the streets. Then we reined him in and he lived with my mother for three years. He needed custodial care. This became my mission: to care for them both emotionally and financially. I did things like managing their household and working to keep my brother away from drugs so he could keep a roof over his head.

Eventually my mother went into a nursing home for her last ten years because she couldn't be left alone with him anymore due to her dementia. She was very resentful for the first three months and I was full of guilt. I worked with her nursing home for her wellbeing as the ever watchful eye. I was glad for her that the staff got to know her when she was still walking and talking so they could bond. I think it helped them give her better care.

My brother couldn't be counted on to care for her and as it turned out he needed his own custodial care, so he was also placed in a facility. He couldn't really help himself, so I became his advocate for the next three years until he died of HIV. He became the primary focus of my life during this time and through my total engagement with the constant drama in his life, I suppose I would say that as his Caregiver he had become my significant other.

Olivia talks about her boyfriend being her central focus

My ex-boyfriend was the central axis of my life for the six years we were together. He died suddenly a year after we split up. He had been a Viet Nam veteran with undiagnosed post traumatic syndrome (PTSD). I didn't really even know what that was at the time. His issues were his suspicions of authority and wrongdoing by others, as well as some guilt and paranoia.

He was very protective of me probably because deep down he felt that I was his mooring. He was deeply concerned for my wellbeing. I gave him structure. If I hadn't cared for him the way I did he would probably have lost all motivation to do things, be social or manage his hygiene.

I didn't feel restricted in my own life because I accepted the way he was and integrated it into our relationship. His care was so much less complicated when compared to what I had done for my brother that I also felt freer as a person while I was with him.

He was an explosive personality. It helped that I didn't try to change him or tell him he was wrong in his views. It was a huge task for me to walk this narrow path with him, and it took all I had to hold myself together for as long as I did.

Olivia talks about her lifelong commitment to her older brother and how during his final years he became the pivotal point in her life

My older brother was seventeen years older than me and had been institutionalized because of his Schizophrenia for as long as I can remember. As an adult I would visit him a couple of times a month and I became completely responsible for him once my parents weren't able to do it anymore.

He became the central axis in my life as he aged because along with his mental illness he now was having the health issues that any senior citizen might expect to have. He required nursing care, but the nursing homes weren't equipped to handle his mental illness. His medical file was huge and it was almost impossible to absorb all the details, so they resorted to medicating him. None of the nursing homes had an official psych ward. I would get calls almost monthly that he was being disruptive, and I would try to reason with him or change the floor he was on. I'd add that the staff has a tough job and many were very helpful in finding even temporary solutions.

We had a strong relationship during those years even though he wasn't able to speak. He was very protective and possessive of me. During my visits he didn't want anyone else to talk to me or interact with us. This was demonstrated with non verbal gestures.

He ultimately ended up moving from home to home due to his behavioral issues. This was very confusing and disruptive for him. He couldn't communicate his needs, so along with caring for him, I also befriended the staff at each location. I hoped that this might improve his care. Towards the end of his life we were really in crisis mode and I became totally devoted to his care until he died.

Musings on Mayeroff:
We develop and find our own identity as we help our significant others to flourish.[80]

Author's reflections:
No person is an island. We become who we are through our interactions with others. We are described as daughters, sons, mothers, fathers, sisters, brothers and a whole host of more distant relations. Most often our family members are the people who we will eventually take care of, or they will eventually take care of us.

Beyond those we are related to by birth, we also enjoy watching our friends grow and flourish into fully engaged adults. Through long conversations on the phone, weekend sleep overs, sharing summer camp memories, all the stuff of satisfying friendships, we become proud to have been a part of their lives. It is especially rewarding when we know we have played a part in our friends' growth. In the end it makes us who we are.

And of course we can't forget those important loves that many of us have found in our spouse, or our life partner. Often these are the relationships that we feel connected to the most. The daily contact, the shared experiences, the common concerns all add to the depth of these significant relationships. In the average person's mind the term "significant other" normally would refer to these relationships.

Does helping those who are significant to you flourish figure into your definition of yourself?

Barbara talks about how she sees herself as she watches her children grow up

I think of my two children as celebrities, and I love being connected to them as their mother. My husband's last dying word was "jackpot" in relation to them. My son has such accomplishments and such dimension.

My daughter is the entire package. She's smart, beautiful, self-reliant, introspective, intuitive, has self-knowledge and perspective. And wow, I'm her mother! I get to see all of this accomplishment up close. I suppose I have allowed her to flourish, but it feels so natural that I hardly noticed I did anything.

Olivia talks about how those she cared for flourished in different ways and how she feels about herself as a result

I do feel that all of the people I cared for flourished to the extent that they could due to my care. I can also tell you that their lives would have been very troubled had I not been there for them. It makes me feel good to have been able to do this for others.

My ex-boyfriend became more trusting due to my care, and as a result his social world expanded greatly. He was very intelligent and well-read but he still felt awkward around others. Before he met me he had projected a tough exterior that put people off. After a time of being together we were able to travel with other couples which would have been impossible for him on his own due to his anger issues. These interactions allowed him to have a much more normal life.

With my two brothers I really was their advocate. I created a safe environment for them. Through my love and concern for them I was able to get them through their fears because I could really sympathize with what they were experiencing. I felt fortunate in my life and I saw them as less fortunate in theirs. I wanted to help improve their situation and I feared what might happen if I didn't step in. It made me feel good to help since I'm a bit of a people pleaser.

When I think about how my friends might describe me, I think they might use words such as kind, thoughtful, "the nicest person I know." I would like others to also think that I acted from my heart more than from my head when I cared for the people who were central in my life. That's the truth of how I feel about myself.

Musings on Mayeroff:
We are "on call" as we make ourselves available to address the needs of the significant person we are caring for.[81]

Author's reflections:
Just telling our loved ones that we miss them and wish they lived closer isn't the same as being truly "on call." Friends who make no effort to spend time together, or families that haven't spent time together to build common memories or traditions, don't fit the criterion of making themselves available for the other.

Having significant others in our lives requires more from us. To truly care for someone at this level requires commitment and action. When we see that our loved one needs us and then make sure we are physically, emotionally and spiritually available for them, we have made a deep connection to this world of caring and to our significant other.

How available do you have to be in order to care for your significant other?

Barbara talks about being available for her children as a single parent

Since my husband died everything about my life is now involved with my children. My personal life is altered and no longer a priority. The house is turned upside down during ski season so I can give my kids the life that my husband and I together would have wanted for them. The laundry is impossible to catch up with because we all would rather do something fun. I gave up any sense of order around the house.

Olivia talks about her availability for her middle brother

With my middle brother I was always available for him. I was on a mission to get everything done, keep it all together, and fit it all in. At first I did what I had to do during the evenings and on weekends. As things got worse I took a lot of time off from work until finally I even took a six week leave of absence to care for him. Things have to get done and who's going to do it? I had to keep things functioning and moving along. He was my primary focus at the time and I even felt that he expected me to make myself always available to help solve his problems.

Taking care of him took a lot of effort. I wasn't able to sleep much and being so exhausted made me feel emotionally like I was on automatic pilot much of the time.

210 When the Voiceless Sing

Chapter 27

Finding meaning in a life well-lived

Author's reflections:
The translation of the title of the legendary French songstress Edith Piaf's most famous song goes like this: "No, I don't regret anything." When we actually live the life that we worked hard to create, everything flows. We find ourselves meeting the right people, having opportunities open up, and ultimately our challenges are met.

When we achieve that life well-lived there is no gap between our meaning and purpose and how they unfold along our path. An example would be when a young adult decides that helping refugees become more comfortable in their new country is what gives them meaning in their life, their purpose becomes all the ways that they find to do this, teaching a new language, helping with housing and finances, bridging cultural differences. Everything on this path now relates to their meaning and purpose.

In the same way a non-profit organization has a mission statement. It is a way of expressing the meaning that the organization has for existing and the purpose is everything it does to achieve its mission. When their members accomplish their meaning and purpose there is nothing to regret in this life well-lived.

Do you feel in sync with who you are and how you are living?

Joe M. talks about being in sync with himself but needing more time to be in sync with how he is living

I'm the same person that I've always been. I think I feel in sync with myself. I have found my meaning in helping others. I don't think I need to do anything differently than I've done all my life. The only difference now is that I don't have a companion since my wife died.

I do relate to others and still try to help them, but my fear is that I might want to go deeper into a new relationship and that brings guilt along with the fear. It's a fear of getting closer to someone new but beyond that that I would get close and then they too might end up getting sick.

This fear of loss is left over from caring for my wife with her cancer and then ultimately losing her. I'm still not over the trauma of that. This is a fear I have from morning to night. How would I handle someone else getting sick and dying or would I be able to handle it? Would it end up the same way as before? These are huge, huge, scary questions.

Christie talks about being in sync with how she is living

Yes, I feel like I have found a rhythm for my life that works most of the time. Because I am involved in so many activities and have found my passions in different areas of expression I sometimes get overwhelmed. I have been known to do a triathlon in the morning and then have a jazz gig in the evening. But this is rare. Usually there is a balance and flow to my life.

Most importantly I feel that I am engaged in activities that fuel my soul and challenge my sense of self. An important aspect of my need has always been to step outside the norm and find something that is uniquely mine. I am in the middle of a big project that will ultimately help hundreds of people. I find the brain storming and problem solving with my team very exciting as we get closer to reaching our goal. We all agree on the meaning that this work gives us and each finds our purpose in what we contribute to the overall project.

In my personal life the blend of my music, sports, dance and acupuncture suits me well. I work on weekends and that is a bit unusual. My free time during the week allows me to enjoy an empty gym, no lines at the bank or supermarket and no traffic when getting around town. I love that I have figured out how to have that kind of quality in my life.

Author's reflections:
When we feel trapped and are always wishing we were somewhere else it is hard to settle into the meaning or purpose in our life or the direction of our path. If we translate this place trap into one of time, then being in the moment is impossible if we are always dreaming about the future or dwelling in the past.

When people indulge in a workaholic lifestyle they often don't have the time or willingness to reflect on the meaning in their lives. If they are lucky they have done this kind of reflecting on the meaning for their life at an earlier point in their lives and now experience themselves living on purpose. Others, however, have never explored why they do what they do and are merely going through the motions of busyness without a connection to their underlying meaning or purpose. These folks often have a vague feeling of emptiness but can't name what it is that is missing for them.

Is there a connection between the direction of your path and the meaning and purpose in your life?

Joe M. talks about his path since his wife died

No, my path has changed dramatically. I don't have any direction at the moment. I do think about what plans I had with my wife but now it seems impossible to do the things we planned because I can't share it with her.

First of all, if I do meet someone new I don't know if they would want the same things that my wife and I wanted with each other. Then again I don't know if I could follow that path with anyone else. I will have to start thinking of a new meaning for myself and if I meet someone new they will add their dreams to mine.

But right now it is all messed up. I have no direct path. I feel like I'm back to being a teenager who is trying to find himself. It's very scary, really scary.

Christie talks about supporting others

I have always come from the school that encourages self-awareness and personal growth as a means of ultimately being able to better care for others. We baby boomers were labeled the "me generation" because we explored Yoga, meditation, psychotherapy, and travel. I never saw these interests as selfish or self-centered. I felt that these pursuits were the basis for a full life. In my mind there also had to be a connection to others and deep relationships for me to have a satisfying and rich life.

I'm not saying that there weren't those baby boomers who were full of themselves and didn't care about others. What I'm saying is that my life would be empty without my relationships.

My background in holistic medicine, meditation and stress reduction all contribute to my friendships and my work. I now find that the purpose of my life is clear and unfolding quickly. I find it important to support my friends as they get older and need more care. They are also finding themselves taking care of others and I support them in that.

Author's reflections:
Knowing and understanding ourselves and taking responsibility for our lives are intertwined with finding our meaning in life. The more we know of ourselves the more we can make good choices about what we are doing on this planet.

How do your self-awareness and your sense of responsibility serve to give you meaning?

Joe M. talks about finding meaning in the midst of his sorrow

I think it is important to be responsible to yourself. In that way I don't want to change. I haven't lost my sense of humor and I think that my kids and my friends appreciate that. I don't bring my sorrows--it's not really depression--to the table with my friends and family.

It doesn't mean that I don't get to a point at family gatherings and holiday affairs where I have to take a few moments to pull myself together. I do. Sometimes it feels like an oasis of emptiness just comes over me.

When I'm alone I reflect on what happened and why it happened. I also spend time wondering what my three kids and my grandchildren are thinking about the new situation in our lives. I wonder if anything I am feeling is being transmitted to them. I am determined that we should all get through this tough time and rebuild our lives holding my wife's memory in our hearts. It is how I find meaning but it is a bumpy road we must navigate as a family.

Joe M. talks about his responsibilities for keeping his family strong

We have had conversations about how my kids miss my wife. Her loss has made us closer and keeping her memory alive for the grandkids has given us meaning to our lives and reason to go on. My four year-old grandchild wants to put special things at "nanny's place", the gravesite. We had a christening a few weeks ago and my daughter gave me a basket of fresh flowers to take to the cemetery. My granddaughter put them on her grave and said a prayer.

I know that my kids are having a hard time dealing with the loss. They used to call my wife every day and ask about cooking and other things in their lives. I still talk to them every day but it's just not the same.

I don't have the same ability as my wife to make occasions special, like birthdays. She had a knack where she could walk into a store and find some silly thing that was just so thoughtful. It's hard without her but we are determined to keep our family strong and united.

Christie talks about her self-awareness becoming her meaning

It has been important for me to be aware of my grieving process. I lost my husband 4 years ago and spent 8 years caring for him. I realize that jumping back into that world of memories can be difficult at times and joyful at others. Thinking about playing music with my husband brings a smile to my face but thinking about his illness and how much we lost makes me sad. This is the emotional roller coaster that everyone dealing with Caregiving refers to.

I tend to meet others who are going down similar paths. I feel it is my responsibility to listen to their stories and give comfort when I can. It does seem to give me some sort of meaning to know I can listen and share experiences. I have realized however, that after other people share their stories of loss and grieving with me, I need to let go of what they shared. Otherwise my heart will continue to break with the stories I hear. So far I have been able to separate myself from the experiences of others as I go about the rest of my life.

Author's reflections:
It turns out that just by its very nature the meaning in our lives has to involve some sort of caring. Caring about our path, our interests, our loved ones, is also completely intertwined with our purpose for why we do what we do. Trying to find something or someone to serve as our meaning and a guide for our purpose is basically impossible without this idea of caring.

Is there anything in your life that is important to you in which caring isn't a major factor?

Joe M. talks about caring replacing competition in his life

I don't really know. I can see things changing for me. What I thought was caring may have been an earlier passion for competition. I seem to care less for my old interests generally since my wife passed away. I also feel that I've mellowed as I've aged. I haven't had to prove anything to anybody and I have felt that way since before her illness. I no longer have to be the best at this or that. Now I really enjoy being with people more.

If my golf game is good it's good and if it isn't it isn't. I enjoy sharing things with my friends such as the Rotary lunches with all the good natured teasing. Bottom line: I've lost my need to compete with others. I do seem to care more about the people in my life now that I know we won't always have each other.

Christie talks about the place that caring has in her life

There is nothing in my life that doesn't involve caring. I care for my music, my sports, my dancing, my interests in science, health and spirituality. My acupuncture clients allow me to be involved in their growth as I care for them. Most of my friends are on a path towards growth and self-awareness and I care deeply for their happiness.

There have been activities that I have suspended because I wasn't experiencing my growth or the growth of the project. I started a music collaborative several years ago but rather than the music being the driving force, I experienced fear from my collaborators. They worried about being left out or not being chosen to play on a particular night. A more formal structure may have worked better, but I was in no frame of mind to start this project over again at the time.

As a result of trying to improve my collaborations in other areas I continue to seek out the most open-hearted partners and the most inclusive projects. If caring for our collective goal isn't top of the list for myself or the people I am working with, then I look elsewhere.

Musings on Mayeroff:
We continuously find meaning as we live our lives in a way that never becomes fixed or static.[82]

Author's reflections:
We often equate finding the meaning in our lives with setting goals for ourselves. But then what happens when we reach our goals? Many people have trouble in their retirement years finding the next thing to get excited about. When the meaning in our lives has revolved around our Caregiving there is also a need for reevaluating our goals once this role comes to an end. If we are lucky our meaning in life carries over to our new projects and relationships but sometimes we need to find a new meaning in life and start over with a new purpose to propel us forward.

Do you still feel like there is more to learn, and that you are continually discovering the elements that make up your purpose in life?

Joe M. talks about himself

I don't really feel like I want to learn something new in my life.... I mostly want to spend time with the people I love. I suppose you could say my meaning in life is that I want to learn more about the people I love, especially my grandchildren. I do want to hear about their achievements and how they are developing. This gives me a purpose in my life and a reason to stay involved in our family's activities. In terms of my friends, I hope they stay healthy and can enjoy what life brings to them and that I'll be able to spend quality time with them for many years to come.

Christie talks about having more to learn

There is always more to learn about people. I have been letting my relationships guide my direction. I know I want to help others and as I meet new people we explore different ideas for how best to accomplish this.

I try to use my creative abilities and my ability to improvise that I have developed through years of playing jazz to think about ways to help other people find solutions to their problems. I'm always walking through different scenarios with my friends to brain storm ways of moving forward in their lives. I do the same thing with my acupuncture clients. It is very satisfying for me to see others grow and move ahead in their lives. When I have no effect on someone who is stuck in a mess I feel unfulfilled and frustrated. I'm aware that my purpose seems to be some kind of facilitator for people who are ready to push forward in their lives. I'm a good coach for them. Their excitement becomes my excitement.

Musings on Mayeroff:
Caring is primary in our life. The meaning in our life comes as a result of our living a life purpose centered on caring for others.[83]

Author's reflections:
Many books have been written about passion and finding something to be passionate about. Passion is often presented as the highest form of involvement in art, music, nature and relationships. Is finding our passion in life the only way to find meaning?

Many people care but fewer are capable of being so passionate. This is not a failing. Caring is ubiquitous among people, available to most and can happen quietly without much drama. It can be sweet and even mellow. It may not get much attention, but caring and especially Caregiving can be the most important aspect of our lives. Many a life has probably been saved by simply caring and being cared for because of the meaning that it brought to these relationships.

How does Caregiving become a central theme in your life?

Joe M. talks about whether Caregiving is a central theme in his life

I do think that Caregiving is very rewarding and that probably anyone can do it. It could be a central theme for some but doesn't have to be. I do believe that a person who is called on to become a Caregiver wouldn't be very happy to not take it on, so my suggestion would be to get involved wholeheartedly when asked.

I don't think the idea of caring being a central theme is just reserved for Caregiving. I think with everyone it is important to care for and about others and their feelings. It's nice to let people know that you care for them and are willing to back it up with action. Just caring about them isn't enough. Keeping in touch is important to me, especially with people I have known all my life. I like to give them a call.

I still have a tremendous relationship with my wife's brothers and their families. They relate to me at the same time that they miss their kid sister. This is a paramount theme, for me to have them all to care for and they return the care. Every week they call and they always include me in everything. They stay close to me and we all do things together.

Christie talks about her work with supporting other Caregivers

I seem to meet Caregivers wherever I go now. I just have to start talking to someone and before I know it they are telling me their story. It feels good having a central theme and it feels like everything makes sense now.

In the midst of the greatest loss of my life I have gained a real empathy for others both in their Caregiving and the loss that sometimes follows. It is almost like a secret society for all of us. I find myself off in the corner with someone at a party or talking to my fellow musicians about the health issues of their family or friends. Instead of running away from it I find that the listening gives me meaning where I can find gratitude for all I still have and for what I have been through because now I can help others in similar circumstances and this gives me a purpose. It all seems to flow for me.

Section F

What describes a life built around caring?

What you receive when you care:

So far we have covered the many aspects of what caring and Caregiving are. For the rest of the book we will be looking primarily at what the Caregiver receives from their experience. We'll look at their new ways of being in the world, new themes and motivations that drive them and major life decisions that all come out of their Caregiving experience.

In addition to the benefits of the direct experience of Caregiving we'll also look at the way life unfolds for the Caregiver who no longer has this role due to recovery of the patient, some kind of transition such as change in location or move to a facility, health issues of the Caregiver or for many the end comes with the death of the person they were caring for. As we will see there is no way to go on with one's life without the experience of Caregiving having a great impact on one's view of the world and on how these Caregivers have chosen to move forward in their lives. Each is unique but all were deeply affected by their role and their experience of Caregiving.

Chapter a

Basic Certainty

Musings on Mayeroff:
As we engage fully with meaning in our life we are nourished and carried along our life's path as we live our values. Our certainty and security come from our full involvement in this path.

   This statement of our values, to care when we are called upon, comes with how we live them. When we are entrusted with the very being of another we can experience a true sense of belonging to our world. As others trust us to live our values and care for their needs, we have a general sense of contentment and belonging on the path we have chosen.[84]

Author's reflections:
There are millions of people who have discovered the joys of caring for others. Many of these people care informally for family members or neighbors while others have decided to join the ranks of the helping professions by receiving formal training and a salary.

   There are also hundreds of non-profit organizations with caring missions and loyal employees who are fully committed to the values of the group. They often aren't paid as much as they might be in the for-profit world, but for these employees, the rewards of being devoted to others, are far superior to a larger paycheck.

   Some of the more successful organizations become like a family for their employees and there is a real sense of belonging for everyone involved. That's one of the main reasons that many non-profits are also able to attract hundreds of volunteers who work diligently without any pay at all.

   When people discover the joys of living in alignment with their values they experience the unity between their inner and outer goals. This unity keeps them energized and excited about the path they have chosen in life.

Are your values different now since you became a Caregiver?

Barb talks about how her values inform her life and her Caregiving

My life and my values are in sync with each other. It's important to me that I live this way. If you know how you want to treat people and you know what your values are, there's a comfort in that. There is no difference in how I care for my mother and how I care for my friends and clients. Trust, devotion and loyalty are all the same for me no matter who I am relating to. Since becoming more of a Caregiver for my mother my values have only deepened, not changed.

Christie talks about how her values came into her Caregiving

I don't think there was much difference in my life before Caregiving. I valued creativity, curiosity and originality and I put all of that into overdrive during my years as a Caregiver. I think my values saved me, actually.

There was probably a greater emphasis on the idea of "other" now. I had never been put to the test to such a degree before this. How much could I care for another? Was I selfish at core or could I grow into this role? My strength was also tested against a powerful opponent, the ravages of Alzheimer's disease. Thankfully I rose to the occasion and was mostly able to care for my husband with an open heart.

Author's reflections:
There are many things that substitute for basic certainty. We sometimes think if we just acquire enough information or find the truth in one situation we'll experience certainty. In actuality our search for knowledge or revelations about life's truths often leaves us more uncertain, and we are left asking more questions or seeking more information.

Sometimes as we search for certainty about how we are living our lives, we decide to take someone else's word as truth. We cling to an authority figure and their beliefs in hope of finding certainty for ourselves. We might choose to go along with what our parents wanted for us, for example, or what a favorite coach recommends. But, if we haven't come to these beliefs for ourselves, if they don't ring true to us, then basic certainty will not come to us. Of the utmost importance in finding certainty is to be able to look deeply into ourselves and our past experiences; we need to be honest and open with ourselves and introspective at the same time.

Has your Caregiving given you a feeling of certainty?

Barb talks about finding certainty in her volunteer work

I wasn't certain at first what being a volunteer Caregiver Coach for the county would be like or if I would be good at it or even enjoy it. We had our official training and our recommended guidelines but I didn't have the experience yet of working with a Family Caregiver. Once I started I realized that my own style came out and that helped me to feel like I was doing something important to help this other person. There was no way the training could give us this kind of certainty. So really, it seems that the personal experience in the field is what creates the certainty in a particular role over time not the training or the certification beforehand.

I can imagine where certainty could be challenged or reinforced by a particular situation as it changes. Dealing with different personalities brings out different facets of who we are. Coaching isn't a static state so depending on the Caregiver's situation and personality the coach's feeling of certainty will be either reinforced or challenged during each session.

Christie talks about finding certainty in caring for her husband and herself

I've run two ultra-marathons in my life. I had lots of advice before the race and others had shared their experiences with me but it was up to me to get out there and do this thing I had committed to.

Aside from the pain and exhilaration, the strongest memory I have of those two days was that I didn't have to do anything else except run all day. I'm not sure whether the lay person can appreciate my joy in the clarity of this singular activity. No distractions, no things to remember about my schedule, no meetings to arrange, no people to call. Just run. I was younger so the thought that I might get injured and that could interrupt my run didn't occur to me. I just ran.

Thinking back to my 8 years of Caregiving I can say that this feeling of certainty returned. I was continually guided by what was needed at each juncture and the required decisions were clear.

I could leave my husband alone in the beginning but once I couldn't I didn't. At first he could entertain himself and stay busy and then he couldn't. I then became the social director and didn't fight the inevitable progression of the Alzheimer's. There were doctors, tests, and opinions. There was research and more opinions. I just let it wash over me and still felt solid in the task at hand.

Alzheimer's doesn't give a lot of leeway. I was told the best medicine was keeping my husband calm and so that's what I did. Of course I'm human and it didn't always go well, but I was clear in the goal to reduce his stress levels.

I also developed a certainty about my own health, stress levels and fitness. I had been a camp counselor in a prestigious New York City day camp for seven weeks in the mid-eighties. It only lasted seven weeks, but due to my two assistants' frequent illnesses, I often was alone with the entire group of 30 three year olds. I remember discovering Maalox Plus for my stressed out digestion. My state of mind at the end of the seven weeks was not pretty. I was burnt out.

There have been other jobs that I've had that ended in the same way with burn out. Since I knew enough about Alzheimer's to know that the person can live with it over many years I knew that this was no time to revisit the state of burn out. I know enough about stress to know that it doesn't only harm those with Alzheimer's. Their Caregivers can also suffer so I knew I needed to keep my stress levels manageable as well.

If this meant taking the extra time and energy to pack us both up for the gym, or pack us up for a picnic at a jazz event, or pack us both up for a jam session in town, I did it. Again there was a certainty that all these steps were important to keep both of us sane and healthy for the long haul.

Musings on Mayeroff:
Finding stability in organizing our lives around our caring helps us withstand inner turmoil, stress and other difficulties in our day-to-

day experiences. We can even be strengthened by these challenges.[86]

Author's reflections:
Certainty cannot be accomplished by the denial of anything negative. This is especially true when we are involved personally. Denial of the progression of a disease, denial of the certainty of death, denial of difficult relationships, denial of financial or legal issues.... None of these denials creates true certainty in our lives. We cannot push all of our perils aside and replace them with a pseudo-calm. Certainty comes with our handling these challenges and responsibilities.

Musings on Mayeroff:
Life becomes simple when it revolves around our caring. The clutter disappears and our ability to focus on what is really important to us becomes sharper.[86]

Author's reflections:
There are aspirations in our world that I consider "false gods." The desire for status is one of these.

My grandmother grew up outside the walls of a wealthy estate. Her father was the church musician. Until she was a certain age she got to play with the rich daughter on the estate. For the rest of her life she tried to gain the status the rich little girl that she had played with enjoyed. Even though she was a successful classical musician, she believed it would make her happy to walk among the wealthy. I saw how it kept her longing for a world she would never achieve and how dissatisfied she was in the world she actually occupied.

Surrounding ourselves with material things is another "false god." We think that having more things will make us happy, but we are actually shrinking the space and opportunities we have available to us. The excess dulls us and we have trouble maximizing our potential and choosing the best options because clutter gets in the way.

Caregiving allows us to organize our lives around something real, the person who needs us. Even when the relationship is a difficult one, we know what we have to do and we do it. There is no time to think of status. Clutter makes what is already challenging almost impossible. It becomes important to stay organized and clear about what really matters. This is the basic certainty of purpose that helps us experience our true character.

Has the underlying caring and love helped sustain you when the going gets rough?

Barb talks about the process of losing her dad

My dad had an aneurysm that they told him could burst at any time. Every time my dad would talk about his vulnerability he would talk about not knowing how long he would be around. It was hard for me because I could really feel his fear and anxiety and of course I never knew when I left him whether I would ever see him again. Even though I loved him very much the fear was also very strong.

Love can be all around you and it can sustain you but there was still a feeling of impending loss. Even though my dad eventually did die, I still have my mother here and it feels like my dad is still with us because we talk about him all the time. So ultimately the love continues.

Christie talks about the love that sustained her when things got rough with her husband's illness

I was very lucky that my husband and I had a great relationship before his Alzheimer's began. The things that came up because we were different people didn't interfere with the love we had for each other. I accepted his workaholic lifestyle and he accepted my need to be more social and travel.

Once he started a steeper decline into the Alzheimer's, I had to make all sorts of arrangements. I think our underlying love definitely pushed me along. He was always happy to see me, showed me how much he loved me. He had turned into a sweet, gentle guy who cried at movies.

Our love helped me the most later on in the disease progression when I was tired and had started getting less patient and more irritable. He was very sharp about detecting my moods and facial expressions long after he could no longer put a sentence together. I could see that he was trying to solve my problems but didn't have a clue how to go about it. I usually softened as I watched his fumbling efforts to cheer me up.

Author's reflections:
What is the best kept secret of all time? And the answer is.... It feels good to be needed. Our species along with most other species do better when we live interdependently. When we care for others, mentor them, cheer them on, train them, love them, they grow to trust and depend on us for these things, and it feels good to us.

Not being needed may feel like freedom at first but at some point that freedom loses its luster. Not being needed feels more like a boat being tossed around on a rough sea. When that happens there is no direction that really matters. Caring helps us find our direction and set the course of our lives.

Does being needed give you direction?

Barb talks about feeling needed

I'm a relationship person in terms of my family, my work and my friends. I enjoy my own time and having my own space as well. It's not so much about having direction but more about experiencing the satisfaction when I can help someone with specific needs that they have. I'm not looking for a thank you when someone is in a crisis. It feels good when after the crisis has passed the person can talk about what they got out of my caring for them.

Christie talks about feeling needed

Yes, I enjoy it when people need me and count on me. It motivates me to be a better person and makes me feel focused and grounded.

The only time I don't enjoy it is when the other person is so needy that they aren't doing their own growing and developing. I start to feel claustrophobic. I like to see the fruits of my labor as others blossom into the fullness of their human potential. When this happens there seems to be a clarity in my giving, a direction for my focus and a certainty to my caring.

Chapter b
Living life is enough

Musings on Mayeroff:
Staying in the moment of our experience is life's true reward, more gratifying than that storied pot of gold said to be beckoning us at the end of an arduous road paved with deeds to accomplish.[87]

Author's reflections:
Eastern religions remind us to "live in the moment." In the West we seem to always need to be somewhere or to be accomplishing something. The New Age joke is that we have become human doings instead of human beings.

In Caregiving this becomes especially important because sometimes the present moment is all we can handle. When we worry too much about the future or long for the past, we can easily become overwhelmed or anxious. In addition, by worrying about the future or longing to have had a better past, we are actually missing the emotional and spiritual experience of being able to reflect on the path that we are presently travelling down with all its rewards and challenges.

What does living in the moment bring you?

Toni talks about living as she engages in her own path

I am certainly not the Buddha; I don't enjoy cleaning! Instead, I enjoy and nurture others through conversation rather than cooking, let's say. When I'm involved with others there is always an element of surprise, and as a musician I crave that. If you mean routines by the "living in the moment" the actual routines of life bore me. I prefer to be directly engaged in my relationships, experiencing nature or creating my music. I think of all of this as my living in the moment.

I do understand the necessity of routines for health, like needing a certain diet to stay healthy. That doesn't mean I can follow it myself. I'm like my brother in that way. Even when I know something is going to help me stay healthy for the future I'll just do what I feel like doing in the present rather than change.

As a teacher I know that routines are important so living in the moment without routines isn't usually possible. When I don't have a routine at school the kids are thrown off. It's hard for me because I don't like routine and just can't do certain things again and again. I prefer to improvise and be creative with the students by living spontaneously in the moment.

Do you enjoy living in the moment or do you feel pressure that you need to focus on the future by working to reach your goals?

Keith talks about taking over his family business

When I was younger I was much more goal oriented. Before this journey of caring for my two sons began I had the idea that I would be the richest man in town by the age of thirty. I had two businesses before my mid-twenties. I failed at the second business and that changed me. After that I came into the family business just to help my dad out. He didn't want to bring anyone else into the business but his partner, my uncle, got sick and died three months later of pancreatic cancer. My dad had open heart surgery a few months after that so he asked if I would help him. He had never asked me for anything before. I was an accountant and had just sold a business so I had some time to give him.

I brought my ambition and being goal oriented to the business which had grown old and stale as my dad aged. I thought we could find more customers and I had a lot of ideas and goals for the future of the business. My whole family encouraged me and would tell me that everything I touched would turn to gold. My cousin came into the business a bit later.

We built up the business and I bought him out about fifteen years ago. Even back then, soon after I came into the business, I realized that it no longer meant that much to me on a personal level. I was more involved as a parent in my children's lives and I felt that I needed to support my wife on an emotional level. I didn't want to miss the important things in my family and enjoying their moments in sports or over dinner were more important to me by then. The business was becoming just a job.

I now realize that we'll always have ups and downs in the business cycle because of trends and styles in gardens and stone work, which is what we do. It doesn't have much to do with me so setting goals isn't really necessary. Right now I could walk away from the business without much trouble. It's nice that it is successful and I do feel generally proud but I'm more involved in trying to find moments to enjoy life with my family outside of work.

Toni talks about her goals and what she enjoys

When I'm working I try to get my work done quickly so that then I can be free to do whatever it is I truly want to do. My goal is to get to that open time where I have no goals and can be free to explore and experience spontaneously.

I consider that freedom as the time that I'm on my journey. I never know what that will be in any given moment but my intention is to stay present to whatever I find. I don't like having set things that I have to do outside of my job.

Musings on Mayeroff:
Being in the moment is central and sufficient; now, our whole existence becomes satisfying, and we no longer need to look elsewhere for fulfillment.[88]

Author's reflections:
One of the things we often find ourselves doing is judging ourselves and how we live our lives instead of simply living and experiencing. Feeling rushed or bored are good examples of how we judge ourselves because either feeling implies that we aren't content with how we are living. In being judgmental, we may feel that the best is yet to come and the now isn't good enough for us.

If we are looking for something that always seems to elude us we need to check on whether our goals are realistic anymore. Trying to have the "good old days" return is an example of an unrealistic goal. We need to be watchful of when we start to feel that our only choice is to endure the unpleasantness we now find, as we quietly long for the days of the past. A change in our perspective may be the antidote to help us find purpose and meaning in our daily tasks.

When things are missing from our expectations the whole Caregiving relationship can turn sour, and unless we know what's happening, it is difficult to fix things and get back on track. On the other hand, if we can switch gears to experience and make things happen in the moment, we may find a more satisfying way to live. Instead of judging and looking elsewhere we may be able to find everything we need in the rich landscape of the path we are already on. We just have to look.

What happens when you feel disappointed in life? Describe your feelings.

Keith talks about feeling his disappointments

When I am disappointed I get what I would call melancholy. It doesn't happen when I'm busy at work. It's mostly the quieter days when it starts to sink in. Maybe a weekend, a Sunday afternoon, or a gray day is when I feel it. I can have a really down day depending on what's going on with the kids or how my wife is feeling and sometimes it's about work if a deal falls through.... I'm grateful when a new day starts so I can get back into a routine again.

I find that when I'm in that kind of mood exercise really helps. I walk everyday on the treadmill or outside and I find that that relieves a lot of the stress.

Toni talks about being disappointed in a co-worker

When I'm disappointed I feel very hurt. There was a teacher at school who told everyone that I put one of my students in her class because he was naughty and I couldn't control him. That really hurt my feelings. I eventually told her that the reason I gave her that child was not to make her life more difficult but that I thought she could confirm my assessment of him to his parents. They might believe our suggestions for him if two of us were telling them the same thing.

Now that she understands my motives she takes care of me at school. I told her that I don't understand how the fact that we had worked together for twelve years and watched out for each other as a team didn't count more with her. That was my disappointment.

Do you feel rushed or bored by life or content with your path?

Keith talks about feeling rushed

Sometimes it feels rushed. I think as I've gotten older I'm more involved in a lot of organizations and my life is generally more complicated. Half the calls I get during the day aren't related to my business. Sometimes it's tenants or people needing me to do things. I get overwhelmed sometimes. I wish I had the time to feel bored.

Toni talks about feeling a variety of things depending on the situation

Work is a combination of rushed and bored. The rest of my life is mostly mellow and I'm content. I don't interact with the world that much so the people that I choose to interact with are relaxing to me.

My life has variety. Sometimes it's boring other times it is interesting, sometimes it's good, sometimes it's fast and sometimes it is slow paced.

Do you wish you were elsewhere or are you content in your life?

Keith talks about having dreams and also being content

I've always wanted to be a missionary. I get really jealous when I hear about the Rotarians that travel and help out in faraway places with dentistry, polio vaccines or recovery from disasters. That's all I really want to do now and if I could leave that's what I would do.

This is my dream and at the same time I'm content in my life as it is now. My dreams for a different future don't ruin my satisfaction in the life I am living. I've accepted my responsibilities as my mother's Caregiver and run her house and schedule the aides to come and help. I'm still my sons' Caregiver as they struggle with their addictions and finding their way in the world. People rely on me, even in Rotary as treasurer. I know all about the money and everyone's asking me what they should do about this or that. I also know that people trust me. My wife is always saying that to me. She teases me and says I should start a hedge fund because people trust me so much. All of these connections are very fulfilling to me as a caring human being.

Keith talks about his sister-in-law's acceptance of her situation

My wife's sister was on the phone last week. She lives in Florida and has a good job in city planning. Her husband hardly works except for an occasional bar tending job at night. He is the house husband and stays home to raise the kids.

She was telling me that she has finally been able to accept her situation. She accepts that things probably won't change. They'll have their two vacations a year and live off of her salary. They'll lease their car and make the payments.

We were talking about how much easier life gets when you can finally accept your situation and stop wishing you were someone or somewhere else all the time.

Toni talks about finding peace

I'm content in my life. I can't think of anything I'd change. I wasn't always like that. I have grown into a peaceful relationship with the here and now.

Musings on Mayeroff:
When caring in all its many aspects is done well, there is no limit placed on it. A caring without limits is constantly being renewed, and offers us a deeper experience. It blends into our life's purpose, leading to our satisfaction, growth and fulfillment.[89]

Author's reflections:

Most of the literature on Caregiving is written from the point of view that Caregiving is a major misfortune. The most common view of Caregiving is that it is burdensome, thought of as exhausting, sad, traumatic or isolating.

It is time to question this singular point of view. Since many Caregivers don't ever see an alternative, they believe the "common wisdom" and suffer in silence. But what about the others, the Caregivers that are thriving in their role, finding purpose and meaning in their caring? We have been looking at many of their stories in this book.

As former Caregivers start to come together to tell their stories and share in full what their caring meant to them, a new perspective starts to unfold. Many tell of the richness of the Caregiving experience, the depth of the feelings they shared, the intimacy and trust that fortified them. They often took on the role for years and years never running out of steam nor having to hand over their job to others. Many, too, maintained their eagerness to learn and felt that they were growing throughout the experience. Their love fueled them and the caring helped them express their love deeply and fully.

When caring encompasses the factors that help it to work, the Caregiver can focus on its positive outcomes: satisfaction, personal growth, connection to others and a deep understanding of themselves and their capabilities.

Do you feel like you have reached your limits as a Caregiver? Do you think that caring has limits?

Keith talks about his Caregiving not having limits and seeing other Caregivers more clearly

In my opinion Caregiving can't have any limits. You just go until you go. I think you have to accept that too. One day you think you can't take any more and the next day you start all over again.

I do have way more empathy for other Caregivers and I see them going way beyond what I think I might have been able to handle. That's for sure. I see them not giving up or giving in either. I see people in much more difficult situations than mine staying with their Caregiving and finding their rewards in the challenges they are faced with.

When I hear that kids have done bad or violent things I can just feel for what their parents are going through. I also seem to be better able to relate to the struggles of humanity as a whole. I'm no longer as judgmental, even about my enemies. Various group members think they are caring for each other. I can still see the unlimited caring even if the expression is distorted, like in gang murders or tribal warfare.

Toni talks about the limits of her caring for her friend

I had a friend who was a drug addict and needed a lot of love and attention. I ultimately refused to get involved after a while. I told her I didn't have the energy. She ended up committing suicide.

From my previous experiences with Caregiving for my mother, father and brother, where I had no limits to my caring, I realistically knew how much energy it would take to care for her and I didn't have it. It was also something that I didn't want to do again because I didn't think there was any winning in it this time.

I felt that there had really been nothing meaningful that I could have done for her. I could have sat with her for an hour but as soon as I left something could still happen. I could see that she wasn't really ready to change or grow or get significant help.

I loved her very much but I felt that her path was a different path and I couldn't join her there. I also felt that there was nothing I could do that would really make a difference.

Toni talks about not having limits during caring for her family but having boundaries with all others

With my mother, brother and another friend I had no limits in my Caregiving. I was open to wherever I was needed and didn't hold back.

With most other people I feel that their needs are almost toxic to me and I do have limits with them. I have boundaries and I know I can't or won't care for them. I also don't want to be all over the place. It takes its toll to see sorrow every day and you still have to put a smile on your face. Your adrenals get stressed and eventually depleted.

In terms of the path you are on are you still curious, open and growing emotionally the way a child might be?

Keith talks about being curious

Yes, I'm very curious as long as I have the time. I'm curious about how my kids see the world and I am always learning from my grandson. My favorite curiosity is the History Channel. Just like a child I still love learning about the way the world works and why the Mississippi River behaves the way it does for example. How do the levees work and where does all that water go? Anything like that amazes me. Where did all that oil go in the Gulf? That's why I enjoy being around kids who are also curious.

My 4 year old grandchild told us one day that he would like to go to the recycling plant to see what they do with all those bottles his mother puts aside. He wants to see them make something else out of them. I'm looking forward to our field trip with him as much as he is.

Toni talks about losing her curiosity

No I'm not that curious anymore. People think I am. I may have lost some of my inquisitiveness after caring for my mother for so long. I was on hyperdrive with finding out all about her Alzheimer's for so long that I think I just need to rest my mind. There are things I'm interested in for a while but then when I return to them I'm no longer interested in them. I do seem to be curious about new ideas. I don't want to think yesterday's thoughts. I look for the grand old masters to teach me and often they are children.

Some people seem to go overboard in their interests and hobbies. They try to get me involved. That's not for me to be interested in other peoples' interests. I need to find my own way. The smallest thing can bring a smile to my face, as long as it is something that reaches me.

The kids at my school are more inquisitive than I am. I don't question things the way they do. Many of the things in my life are familiar to me. I go over the same terrain and sometimes find new ways of seeing the familiar.

Do you feel like your path is helping you grow?

Keith talks about his own growth

I never think of it in those terms. I am growing from all the things I've had to deal with, but if you gave me a choice I probably wouldn't have chosen this path. It's a tough question. For me to evaluate myself as a parent and ask if I've grown, I don't think I'm a good parent according to my ideals and standards. If you ask me the same question in ten years I might be able to see the growth and the positive things that came out of our situation.

If I look at ten years ago, those were much better times. Our kids were playing sports and the older kids were having their first babies. I almost feel like I've regressed. However, I know I could never have accepted then what I accept now so there's growth in that. If I hadn't learned this skill of acceptance I would have gone mad or I would have had to leave or done something drastic.

Thinking of my wife, we have both grown into the acceptance of our situation. Lots of other couples split up when a mother moves in and we've had both of our mothers to deal with. I accept that my wife and I have different ways of dealing with things. Eventually these situations will pass and I realize underneath our different styles we both want the same thing. We both want what's best for our kids. Sometimes her choices might be best and sometimes mine might be and hopefully it will combine into a good outcome for our two boys.

Toni talks about her own growth

I got a dog and there was growth in that. I'm also reconnecting with friends from an earlier time in my life. I'm growing as I learn how to bring these relationships into my life as it is now. It's fun for me to do this. I see how we can still communicate and understand each other.

I see growth in myself and in a group I belong to. I belong to something called the Circle of Light. It is a way that a group of people can care for each other. It started as a group of four people online. By the time my cousin invited me to join there were fifteen people and now there are thirty members ranging in age from thirty to ninety years old. Most of them are artists or musicians. I didn't know that at first.

How it works is that each day someone is in the center of the circle and they can write about anything they want to and the rest of us support them. We have been there for each other through death, birth, and various transformations.

Suddenly there was a huge growth spurt for the entire group. What happened was that my cousin gave the writings of the group to her students to use as the basis for a video. I was so excited by it all that I could hardly sleep. People were writing wonderful things and even wrote songs. They were really flying. I'm growing because I see all the different ways of creating that the group shares and that the students will capture it all for their project.

Chapter c
Understanding and wonder

Author's reflections:
In this world of experts we often hear about one scientific study or another. The goal of the scientific method, used in modern science, seems to be to uncover truth by carrying out studies in which the investigators control the methodology and the outcomes are predictable.

In the scientific world wonderment and surprise are undervalued. Rather, researchers seem to be looking to solve problems and find answers instead of savoring the unfamiliar. They impose their own limited and rationalized explanations onto their inquiries in search of uniformity and the results they have predetermined to achieve.

When our world is seen filtered more through our rational minds and less with the subtlety of our senses, we become distant from ourselves and personal growth becomes limited. We cut off major ways that information enters our lives, and this makes it harder to learn and experience the world fully.

Valuing equally the understanding and the wonderment in our lives helps us create themes which give us meaning as we engage in life to its fullest, far beyond the purely rational limits we so often impose.

Musings on Mayeroff:
When we live each day practically, in sync with our true meaning, almost magically we attain the wisdom that allows us to discover what we need to flourish and why we are alive.[90]

Author's reflections:
Wisdom evolves over our lifetime. Understanding why we do what we do, how to do the things we do and what is needed to accomplish our goals is all a part of this lifelong learning.

It can be boiled down into three steps. Step one, find a central theme in your life. It could be Caregiving or writing songs, for example. That's the why we are living. Step two, energize this theme in a meaningful way and infuse it with life. Be the best Caregiver that you can, or the best songwriter. That's the how we are living. Step three, learn from this process what is needed for it to blossom like a beautiful, springtime garden. What would feed our hearts for our Caregiving, or what would fuel our creativity for our song writing? That's the what we need for living the meaning of our life.

Do you feel you have attained any understanding and wisdom from your Caregiving? Give some examples of what you now understand.

Claudine talks about discovering a central theme in her life

I understand that we have no control over others. The only thing we can control is our own perspective. From my Caregiving and parenting I learned that it's a waste of energy trying to fight this. Once I learned this fact of life a lot of other things fell into place, so this is really a central theme for me.

Marian understands her self-worth

I understand that I have self-worth and I offer that now in all the ways I am engaged in my life. I learned that I could do what seemed on the surface impossible to do, and I've done it. I learned that I could do more than manage. I created a good life for my husband and myself during the years of his dementia.

Other people say they could never have done what I did. Maybe they could have and maybe not, but I did it and I still feel very proud of myself. It's a very strong feeling I have to this day and it supports me in the work I do in my community and in my relationships with my friends and family.

Musings on Mayeroff:
Caring is the cornerstone of what we value in our own life, and once we can appreciate that, it becomes easy to understand how this is also so in the world outside; everything now seems to fall into place.[91]

Author's reflections:
In the face of all the technology that keeps us isolated in our own little cocoons, listening to our music, or watching TV shows on our iPads, there are movements afoot to change things.

Communities understand that things need to change and are looking for ways to become more livable by making it easier for their citizens to connect to each other. Creating communal gathering sites for seniors, Caregivers, teens and artists brings us all together to share our skills and connect our talents. Intergenerational programing connects older and younger generations to build on each of their strengths. Making learning available for all is another way that communities remain strong and grow resources.

As the idea of caring as a central theme to help us connect to each other becomes more understood, there will be more and more opportunities created to build strong communities as we care for each other.

Do you think the world would benefit if you shared what you understand about caring?

Claudine talks about learning about listening, compassion and acceptance

As I cared for my parents I learned that it is important to be a good listener and to be compassionate in my caring. Being accepting is also important.

I think the world would definitely benefit from these same things that I learned. I truly believe if everyone listened to and accepted each other more and could find it in their hearts to be compassionate towards each other this world would be a much better place.

As a teacher who cares deeply for my students I understand that the education system is already making great strides in their ability to teach compassion compared to when we were in school. They are teaching about inclusion, bullying, and having more open-minded discussions when dealing with peers. Hopefully these lessons will eventually take root in the larger society as these students move into their lives and a more caring society will emerge.

Marian talks about understanding that love and respite are very important for Caregivers

I think the world would benefit by learning some of the same lessons that I learned as I cared for my husband for many years. I learned that if it feels right, it is much better to try to express your love to the person you are caring for. That's the real reason we are all doing this work, hopefully, not because we love the work but because we love the person.

At the same time I now understand that it is important to also try to get some respite from the situation. That was especially important to me during the last stages of my husband's illness. I paid for someone to come in once a week so I could get out of the house for a few hours.

I would usually go to my exercise classes but one time I went to Macy's. I hadn't been to the store in ages. There was a sale and I was enjoying looking through the racks of clothes. Another shopper recognized me and came over to chat but I resented it. She was taking up my precious alone time to shop. I apologized to her and I was surprised that I would feel that way. Looking back I can see how important those breaks were for me.

Musings on Mayeroff:
Wonder comes with creativity. No one can say exactly how creativity happens but it seems to work better when we become more childlike. Children wonder about everything. Wonder is an intrinsic part of life that doesn't need to be dispelled or solved like a problem. There is no special understanding when it comes to something so unfathomable as the many mysteries such as birth, death, beauty and love. There is no need to do more than wonder at our very existence.[92]

Author's reflections:
It's OK that our brains can't comprehend how wondrous life is. A musician can't say why they chose certain notes or why certain melodies make people cry, and that's OK. We are left to wonder at great beauty and heroic acts, for example. There are certainly more than the seven wonders of the

world. These things don't need explanations.

When it comes to wonder there are no secrets that need to be revealed. We can learn about history, how the pyramids were made and why, but it doesn't take away from the wonder we feel at their existence. Awe and appreciation are enough in the presence of such greatness. That is one type of wonder.

Caregiving gives us a front row seat to another type of wonder. This is the type of wonder that happens when we just can't wrap our brains around something. It's the "head scratching" type of wonder.

We are watching life at its most intense when we give care, and many times what we experience is beyond our understanding. We wonder how we do all the things that are required of us; we wonder what will be the outcome, we wonder at the physical processes we are witnessing, and we wonder at the spiritual strength that we call upon when we need it most. In addition, when we face loss, it turns a spotlight on what we still have, and we wonder at that as well.

What does "a world full of wonder" conger up for you?

Claudine talks about finding inner peace as a link to wonder

I think of a non-judgmental world when I think of wonder. I also think that when someone is at peace with themselves and not judging themselves it is easier to experience this wonder. I feel like this is our choice. You can choose to see the negative and the narrow or you can choose to see the beauty and the openness.

Claudine talks about her husband finding wonder in the midst of horror

My husband was part of the cleanup workers at Ground Zero after 9/11. For days and days they were removing the body parts of the people who had died on that day. On one particular day my husband was extremely exhausted. He encountered a dismembered leg with a steel bar going through it. All he saw was a beautiful flower instead of the horror of that image. His mind was protecting him. Images of goodness and evil were both there and he chose the flower. He still talks about how that experience gave him hope and allowed him to continue his work.

Marian talks about finding wonder in art and music

I enjoy the process of doing art but I'm finding it's not easy. I get excited about it in my classes. I also enjoy sharing the challenges of making art with the other people in the class. When I go to museums or exhibits to see other people's art I can see it with a different eye now. I look for the light and negative space. There is so much more I appreciate now in the variety of expressions, the color, the light and the emotion. Art now fills me with a deep awe.

My husband and I used to go the symphony together. I always had a love of classical music from my musician parents. Certain music brings back memories of the concerts they played. After my husband died I decided to take his love of opera and get myself a season subscription. I'm really enjoying it. I feel like it is his gift to me. Since having been a Caregiver I now look at everything more carefully but I don't need to analyze it. I'm finding a wonder in music that I can appreciate more now. I consider it a great luxury.

Musings on Mayeroff:
Wonder comes with the very awareness of our existence and that of the world around us. The mysteries of birth, life, love and death can remain.[93]

Author's reflections:
The term "conscious living" is used in the world of holistic health and in many Eastern religions. At any juncture in our lives we have a choice to "survive" or "get through" our experiences or to grow and learn from our path by heightening our awareness of life's process. Our ability to grow comes from our ability to recall our experiences and to reflect on them.

What can come with this awareness is an overwhelming feeling of incomprehensibility. We can't conceive that stars we may be seeing today are no longer there. The distances in our solar system are too great for us to wrap our brains around. How can things be so far away that its take so, so long for their light to reach our eyes?

The mysteries of birth, life, love and death are there to awe and inspire us. These are the subjects of our art, literature and music. They are not scientific puzzles that need a solution. The mystery can linger and our awareness lets us appreciate and wonder at it all.

What ideas are you happy to contemplate and not fully understand? Is it okay to have mysteries in your life or would you prefer to have explanations for everything?

Claudine talks about having angels she can talk to

After both my parents died I had a strong feeling that I now had someone to talk to directly in the great beyond. I didn't need an explanation for this feeling. I just went along with it. After each of their deaths my parents became my angels and I feel I can still ask them for help. I don't pray anymore but instead I talk to my angels. When I ask for very specific things that I need help with, things start to happen. It can be silly things like parking. I ask my dad to help me with that. Just as I'm about to give up there is a space! I don't try to understand it. I just smile.

My mom had her opinions about my life. When she was alive she would say that I wasn't cut out to be a school administrator. Even after her death it feels like she may have put some obstacle in the way to prevent my promotion to administrator. Again I don't try to fight it or understand it especially.

Maybe in ten years or so I'll know what her plan for me is. I tried going into business, and when that didn't work out all these teaching jobs have suddenly come to me. When will I get it that this is what I am supposed to be doing? My mother seems to know it already!

I'm fine with having mysteries in my life. I don't need explanations for everything. There is probably some reason for natural events and disasters but we just don't know what it is. Why would you have an earthquake and tsunami to cause so much damage? It's a mystery. Science can't explain it fully.

Marian talks about being comfortable with mystery and her faith

I'm OK with having mysteries in my life. I don't need to know who is guiding me or exactly how. In reality I feel like I am a part of it too so I don't need to understand how it all works together. There have been times where I've avoided accidents and it felt like it was beyond my controlling the outcome. I don't need to know specifically what that force was.

I have a deep inner faith and I don't need to understand it or express it verbally. I'm not one of those people who can make up prayers on the spot. This is only in the area of religion for me. I feel like I have a relationship with God and especially the angels and can ask for things I need. My husband and I both felt that we had guardian angels guiding and protecting us. I'm OK with these mysteries.

Musings on Mayeroff:
This ability to wonder at the unknowable gives us a direct experience of being linked to all creation. There is no need to avoid the immensity of the questions of our existence. This is not like the supernatural that only some have access to. We all can deeply know that no matter how skilled, affluent or knowledgeable we are or aren't, at the deepest levels we are all the same.[94]

Author's reflections:
Whenever someone talks about quantum realities I sense that they are talking about the ways that we are all linked to each other. Laws of nature apply equally to the simplest of life forms as well as the most complex of beings.

I also feel this connection when they talk about the tiniest parts of creation, a nano, a neutrino, even an atom. On this level we are all the same. Having a feeling of oneness with all creation is the time honored definition of personal enlightenment.

Psychics, fortune tellers and others who claim to read our thoughts, talk to the dead, and know our futures are not experiencing this oneness with others. Their powers separate them from the rest of us.

Knowing that there is a connection with all of life, to other beings and to all of nature can be the source of our comfort and continued investigation. This context of connection can be how we learn and grow into ourselves.

Did you ever have the sense that universal human truths bring us closer together? How might this play out?

Claudine talks about the common goal to provide for our families

As humans we all have things in common. We all hope for basically the same things. We all want to raise our children in a safe world. We want to be able to feed, dress and educate them. We also want to care for each other during difficult times. This doesn't necessarily bring us closer together when there is no respect for how each of us goes about fulfilling these desires. There often isn't agreement on how to provide for our loved ones and neighbors so we end up fighting over our differences.

We would be better served to focus on our own behaviors to do good in the world and accept that others have different ways of achieving the same things.

Marian talks about the common desire for personal freedom

There is something in our modern times that has inspired people around the world to want their human freedoms. I don't know if we would all agree on what that freedom stands for but it connects us to all be on a path towards gaining some sort of personal freedom.

It might be the new technologies that are creating the desire for freedom. Information and the skills to do something about an oppressive situation may be adding to an ability to rebel against the old and create something new. This might eventually even happen in this country as more people are suffering without jobs or hope for the future. For many people having a decent life means freedom, in this case financial freedom. Others may be thinking of freedom of the press or freedom of expression. These are universal needs that we all hope to achieve.

When I read the paper about countries that are struggling to overcome oppression I feel closer to those on the front lines of the struggle. I don't know if this feeling is stronger in me now that I cared for my husband for so long. I seem to be able to relate to other people's dreams and goals better. I can certainly relate to struggle better now that I experienced my own struggles and overcame my own difficulties.

Musings on Mayeroff:
In living and in contemplating our existence deeply we get to know the worth of our unique contributions to our world and at the same time are humbled by our insignificance when seen in the context of the entire history of our universe.[95]

Author's reflections:
Reflection is something that needs time and quiet. We are living in a noisy fast-paced world. It is hard for many of us to imagine the austere life of

monks during their many hours of meditation. Finding time to reflect is especially difficult for Caregivers.

The rewards are great when we do find the time for reflection or meditation. Our confidence grows as we realize we are unique and our gifts to others are like no one else's contribution. Our time here on earth, including our time as Caregivers, has been influenced in both small and large ways by our unique outlook and energy.

As we contemplate ourselves in relation to the history of the entire universe, we have that view of being a speck of sand or a unique snowflake. This can bring us to an understanding of humility in a way that makes our contribution seem quite small. At the same time, however, we may still see that contribution as an important one.

What do you understand to be your unique contribution to others?

Claudine talks about herself as a listener

I'm a great listener. I use my listening skills at home and in the classroom. I listen to the people I care for, especially my husband and my daughter. They share their worries and their health issues with me.

It's sometimes easier for me to listen to complete strangers. That's because I can feel compassionate due to the fact that I'm not emotionally involved. I don't feel any hurt from the past when I listen to strangers.

Marian talks about her community projects

Now that I finished my Caregiving and parenting roles I can bring that same energy to my neighbors and friends. My gift is that I'm very creative and generous with my efforts. I'll give you just one example but there are many others I could talk about.

When I take on a project like hosting the monthly dinner here at the condominium complex, it's fun for me to add a special flavor and with an extra effort to make it an experience. For example if I've chosen an Italian theme for a romantic Valentine's dinner. I want to create an ambiance for the guests that allows them to feel like they are in Italy. I use decorations, music and special candles in wine bottles and things like that. It's more artistic and fun than the usual dinners we have. I do lots of extra things to help make it special.

Musings on Mayeroff:
Quiet allows us to become more aware of ourselves and the silence around us. We need to make an extra effort in this noisy world to eliminate the distractions that surround us.[96]

Author's reflections:
I like to say that we humans have become entertainment-seeking devices. With our hundreds of TV channels, music downloads, our eReaders with thousands of books, magazines, journals and blogs to choose from and now unlimited instant downloads of our favorite movies, what is becoming of our quiet time?

To change this we would first have to see the benefit in experiencing time away from all our toys, and then we would have to make an extra effort to find some quiet time and space. Caregiving makes finding quiet time even more rare. Of course studies show that meditation and being in an Alpha state of relaxation improve our health, mood and ability to create, but we need to learn this for ourselves.

What we get from this quiet time is a clearer understanding of what the themes of our lives are, and we also have a chance to contemplate the big picture with all its wonder and mystery.

Do you have the time and quiet to contemplate the larger issues in your life and find the wonder in it all?

Claudine talks about taking time for reflection

I'm trying to find the time to reflect. I spend this time asking for help in my life from my angel guides. I try to visualize what I am looking for and the path I am heading down. They say visualizing something specific makes it closer to becoming a reality.

I also reflect on the people in my life and what I want for them - health, satisfaction, clarity and contentment.

Lastly, I love to wonder at the world we are sharing, its beauty and its mystery. Nature is a great comfort to me, and I live in a very beautiful place.

Marian talks about keeping busy rather than reflecting on things

I don't really spend my time thinking about these big picture things. I think I keep myself busy on purpose. That was my initial reaction when my husband died. I may not be ready yet to be more reflective because I haven't reflected on the loss I experienced.

I keep myself busy no matter what. I run around less now because I can't go to my swimming class so I have a block of time. Lots of other things seem to fill up that time. Instead of thinking in the car, I'll put music on the radio.

I do reflect on the things that the teachers bring up in our art class by looking at the art that is all around me. I do this with music too. I suppose that is my reflection time, through wondering at and appreciating the art and music I experience around me.

Chapter d

Autonomy through dependence

Musings on Mayeroff:
Our individuality comes along in part with our achievements and a certain amount of maturity. It isn't there at birth. We experience the freedom to be ourselves in each moment and that hopefully becomes a comfortable way to live.

We grow into having our own autonomous life. It happens as we act on our beliefs and make things happen. Most significantly, our growth into who we are becoming happens as we care for our interests, our expression, our work and especially for the others in our life. Our personal growth goes along with our ability to also take responsibility for this caring.[97]

Author's reflections:
Depending on how we are raised we develop notions about being dependent on others. If dependency is presented as a weakness then, as we mature we may choose to become personally more detached. Many people that we observe as loners are examples of those who, as children, didn't have close friends and as budding adults, never found groups to be a part of and identify with. They may have also been unable to form or maintain strong emotional bonds with family.

Sometimes the excessive need for independence is a rebellion and a need to feel free and unrestrained by others. There's often a related desire to find pleasure without limits or responsibilities. Any thrust towards full maturity is stunted.

The notion of personal freedom is tossed around like a rowboat in high seas. When people are asked about what freedom means to them they often refer instead to the choices they have -- "freedom" to drive a red or a black car, "freedom" to own a gun, "freedom" to say what they think: but these are really choices and don't convey the broad understanding of the word "freedom."

Freedom in its highest form allows us to become who we truly are beyond our everyday choices. It is important to ask if we are living in an environment that allows us to realize this potential and at the same time allows others to realize their potential. Our individual power stays intact as we also allow others the freedom to be themselves and to create a powerful life that they find meaningful and full of purpose and direction.

Sometimes a person prefers to be free from commitments, valuing their independence above all else. Do you know anyone like this?

Julie speaks about when she can feel committed and when she can't

That's me! In a certain way I totally value my independence. I don't want to live with somebody and I don't want an intimate relationship because it would impinge on my independence. I am, however, committed to my friends and family as long as they don't move in. I have experienced a feeling of terror when I've thought that somebody I love might have to move in with me.

Olivia speaks about someone she knows who prefers to be free from commitments

I know someone who prefers to flow through life and isn't interested in commitment at all. They want to feel in control in all situations and they see commitment to others as an obstacle to feeling in control.

Author's reflections:
Many individuals are unable to appreciate their own need to grow and to seek a life of fulfillment. They become stagnant and bored with their choices and don't understand why. They look for excitement outside of themselves and are unable to animate themselves or others from within. Instead of their world getting larger with all sorts of possibilities, it shrinks and things start to feel superficial and meaningless. Life no longer seems hopeful and full of promise.

Sometimes a person seems flat and unable to get excited about anything. They may frequently complain about being bored. Do you know anyone like this?

Julie speaks of her students and her godchild having a flat affect or bored with life

A number of the younger students in the last group I taught had that flat affect. I don't really know what was going on with them and I can't really judge them. If someone I met socially had that flat affect I wouldn't spend any time with them. I need more growth, connection and excitement in my relationships.

    I had a discussion with my godchild about his boredom. I was saying that there's no such thing as something being intrinsically boring. He may be bored but that doesn't mean that the thing in question is boring. The discussion angered him because he couldn't see that it was his reaction that created his boredom.

In terms of other people, most people seem to be filled with too much anxiety these days to feel bored. Boredom has been replaced by restlessness. That may be related to so many people being plugged into technology all the time and focusing on external stimulants. If they didn't have their cell phones, internets and iPods then there would be more boredom, I'm pretty sure.

Olivia speaks about someone she knows who is always bored

I know someone who is bored all the time and it seems to come from the idea that the world owes them something. They don't seem to be able to initiate anything for themselves. They don't have the ability or diversity of imagination to act on a plan so they are always broke. Not being able to afford to acquire the things they think they want then leaves them hopeless and unmotivated. It's a vicious circle.

Musings on Mayeroff:
We are the ones responsible for our lives, and this gives us a sense of direction for what, where and how to initiate our actions. This is an intrinsic aspect of our growth and can't be initiated by others.[98]

Author's reflections:
Modern life, which is fed by modern media, has created a model where competition reigns. In this model there are winners and losers; winners are encouraged to be vindictive and losers are meant to feel humiliated. This approach, when applied to society, spills over into the market place where we are all turned into products competing with one another to be "sold," and we go about packaging ourselves to make us "marketable." We become a trendy commodity branded and poised for the success we may never achieve.

We are promised we'll get a better job, a better relationship, a better lifestyle, but in this way of doing business there are always losers who miss out. We secretly wonder if we'll become one of them in the midst of our hype.

When we choose our direction based on our inner reflections and personal goals, then things become clear. Often our life's purpose is connected to our relationships and our satisfaction comes with our caring for others. A soldier's motivation for serving is more often to care for and defend their fellow soldiers as opposed to the commonly-believed notion that they serve merely to defeat the enemy.

Competition becomes less inviting to those who have found a powerful direction along with strong relationships in their lives. Their inner direction guides them to their purpose in life and their purpose in life guides them to experience true satisfaction in caring for others.

Sometimes a person is very competitive. Do you know what their life is like? Do you think they are happy and have good relationships?

Julie speaks of how competitive her sister's friend was

My sister had a friend for many years. Her personality was competitive and she needed to be in control. I don't think she was happy. She had a terrible relationship with her own family. She tried to control my sister and even when they went on vacations she would always control their activities. I don't think she was capable of having a good relationship where she would let the other person grow and explore. In her controlling everything she had to hold on to tight reins.

Olivia speaks about working in a competitive environment

I work with many competitive people because that is encouraged in our business. I don't think they are happy because in the things they are seeking they don't allow themselves to relax. They always have to go towards what is on the cutting edge of styles and trends. In this external seeking they aren't really being true to themselves. I think it would be hard to be in a relationship with them.

Competition at any cost is probably not good for any of them personally. They leave themselves out on a limb to fall if the wind blows the wrong way. They would be better off building stronger relationships so they would have some cushioning to fall back on if they got into trouble. I think they are so wrapped up in their trendy world that they no longer have a concept of what the rest of the real world is experiencing.

Musings on Mayeroff:
We learn over time to understand ourselves and then we can know what our needs and goals are. Now we are ready to be called on to care for others, to facilitate their growth.[99]

Author's reflections:
As Joseph Campbell expressed it at the end of his life, in looking back on how he had lived it, everything made sense. Life can be viewed as a series of unrelated events or it can be regarded as the intricate weaving of a cloth that connects everything. Life can be lived as a passive journey or there can be a sense of growth and discovery that comes with working actively on things.

In this process of growth we learn about ourselves and how we relate best to others. By actively creating our lives we demonstrate to the world the lessons we have learned concerning how we need to best live on this planet.

Do you know anyone who, if they don't reach their goals immediately, loses interest in continuing on? How does this relate to finding meaning in their life?

Olivia talks about competitive people

I think the same personalities that are competitive are also less patient and want everything yesterday. I think our business world encourages instant gratification and we reward for instant success. Once they reach their financial goals there's nowhere else to go that holds any meaning for them beyond always wanting more stuff.

It would be better to reward for merit over time and include the bigger picture of what one's contributions are to the team. It might foster more cooperation and the young people might become more thoughtful about what's really important in their lives.

Christie talks about a friend preferring daring escapades over working towards long term goals

A few years ago I had gone to a dance class with a friend. We didn't know what to expect but we thought we'd try it out. I immediately knew I had discovered my passion and I've been taking dance classes for the last several years.

My friend ended up being restless and had some trouble with the basics. She already knew how to dance a bit and didn't see any reason to learn more if it was going to be hard or require work.

She enjoys individual events where she can be successful and experience something daring almost immediately. Skydiving, sailing, riding motor cycles all give her the thrills she enjoys. Personal growth which is accomplished by taking on the longer term challenge of learning more and going deeper into a single area doesn't seem to appeal to her.

Musings on Mayeroff:
In caring we are guided by the needs of others in helping them grow and guiding them to learn to care for others, as well as our need to grow within the relationship.[100]

Author's reflections:
They say that no man is an island but what does this really mean? How connected to each other are we really? Is it a coincidence that when someone suffers from depression they often mention not feeling connected to others or that they prefer to be alone for long stretches of time? Which comes first, the isolation that creates the depression or the depression that invites the isolation?

On the other hand most of our happiest memories are those we have shared with others, either events or accomplishments where others cheered us on. Watching others reach their goals gives us a wonderful lift as well. That's why we attend the graduations and weddings of those we love.

Doesn't it make sense then that becoming even more deeply involved over time in the needs of others would bring even greater connection in our relationships as compared to a one day celebration? Becoming more understanding of our own need to grow as we refine our caring to suit their needs may be exactly what we have been seeking.

Watching someone learn and grow in the glow of our caring, may be the key to our own growth and fulfillment. Watching how we blossom through their joy and success can be observed in our reflection of what we hold most dear.

Do you know anyone who finds their meaning by caring for others?

Julie talks about her two caring friends

Every minute of every day 24/7, my friend is caring for others. She works at an arts service organization all day. Then she spends time calling people who live in the poorest areas every single night. She also spends hours on the phone with a colleague's brother who has multiple concerns. Now her mother is in a nursing home on the upper West side of Manhattan and she is always checking on her. She even took care of her client's dog after he passed away.

Our other friend has decided through her religion that she would also do service that involves Caregiving. She works for a different service group and actually lives at the center so this has become her life's mission.

Olivia speaks about herself finding meaning as a Caregiver

I think Caregivers find meaning in what they are doing. I know I did. I don't think that Caregivers get enough respect for being able to put themselves in the shoes of another. That's what they find meaningful.

Their kindness takes over and before they realize what's happening they are in a Caregiving relationship. There are many ways to find meaning in Caregiving and some relationships are more demanding while others are not. Some require longer commitment and more focus while others require less involvement. I see Caregivers all around me, caring for their sisters, parents, children and spouses. Most of them wouldn't trade their role for anything.

Do people who care for others experience great satisfaction?

Julie talks about a friend who defines herself through her caring

My friend is so involved in her Caregiving that I don't even know whether she is satisfied with her efforts. It goes beyond satisfaction. It is her definition of herself.

As a teacher she has always wanted to give to others, since she was a child. Now that she has had a chance to teach acupuncture, it has brought her tremendous satisfaction.

Olivia talks about how Caregivers find satisfaction

Obviously when things go well it is easier to feel satisfied as a Caregiver. When you feel like you are doing a great job it feels like a pat on the back. Why do some people just dive in? Maybe it is the aspect of problem solving, again when things are working you can feel satisfied or proud of yourself. Maybe it is the only way to feel in control of a situation that is in all other ways out of control due to illness or some other difficulty.

It would be nice if someday the outside world would show their appreciation for the daily work that a Caregiver does. Satisfaction is nice but recognition is important too.

Musings on Mayeroff:
To be autonomous we need to care for ourselves, understand ourselves and know what we are reaching for. There isn't a randomness to our autonomy nor is there an unfamiliar feeling to it. We need to know how to satisfy our needs in order to become autonomous.[101]

Author's reflections:
With a certain amount of self-reflection we can usually begin to identify our goals, dreams, desires and what it would take to achieve them. These are the things we grow to become dependent on for our autonomy.

Without this self-awareness we can never be sure we are on the right path towards accomplishing our goals; our choices seem to be made randomly and we tend to go with whatever feels good at the time.

Sometimes there is a feeling that we know what choices we want to be making but we just can't get there. This happens a lot when it comes to caring for ourselves. We know what we need to do but we just can't seem to make the right choices. Sleep, nutrition, exercise, relaxation and good relationships all suffer if we can't make good choices.

As we develop more of a sense of who we are, why we are here and where we are headed, our ability to care for ourselves gets clearer. We start making better choices without all the effort involved with willpower and discipline. Knowing who we are leads us to what we must do and how we should live. We become dependent on this sense of direction and all the choices that have contributed to our growth including our caring.

How does caring unify people's goals and the path they are on?

Olivia talks about how caring has unified her goals

In my case I now bring caring into the work I do and the relationships I have. Caring seeps into everything I do because I think like that now. It's how I treat people by always offering to help them. I also usually have ideas of how to help and because of that others will call upon me. Caring is now the bedrock of who I am in all areas of my life.

How does this unified goal of caring affect the growth of the person they are caring for as well as their own growth?

Julie speaks of her friend's work and her lack of time to reflect on her own growth

My friend's clients are mostly heavily medicated, poor, psychiatric patients of color and then there's the brother of a colleague who is both a genius and completely insane. She probably saved his life and helped him avoid committing suicide a long time ago.

Their quality of life for those she cares for has improved tremendously because of her help. Some of these people were homeless before they met her. She got one client an apartment under Section 8 and this is because she is really good at the bureaucracy that is involved.

In terms of her own life I'm not sure she has attained the type of confidence and feeling of self-worth that you might think would come along with such wonderful work. She may not be having the time to reflect on what it is she is doing and how much goodness she brings to other people's lives or how much she has grown over the years.

Olivia speaks of the growth of the person being cared for as well as the Caregiver

Often the person being cared for may have been stunted in some way or derailed from their original path. A Caregiver is trying to keep them alive with dignity and help them reorient to what their new possibilities are. They might try to keep them engaged in a more positive outlook for their life.

It depends on whether they are caring for someone with an illness or dementia. If they are caring for someone with a fatal illness they may try to offer some kind of relief.

The fact that someone can do all this as a Caregiver helps them grow into a fully connected human being. I know that my Caregiving experiences changed my life. I look at things very differently. I can also sense when someone has never had a Caregiving experience. There's something missing in who they are. I can just tell.

Musings on Mayeroff:
We need to be fully engaged in our lives to feel comfortable with who we are. At the same time we must avoid the ubiquitous pitfalls in our culture that stifle our growth.[102]

Author's reflections:
Finding a passion for things in our lives is a blessing. Most artists and musicians can recall clearly how they found their passion. It might have been a mentor that guided them. It might have been the applause or acknowledgement that they received from others. It might have been a wonderful role model that they one day dreamed of becoming.

People who rescue animals often tell of a menagerie of furry ones that they cared for as a child. Their desire to rescue animals that are in trouble might have started with a favorite pet that helped them through difficult times.

Those who like to read or write find joy in the language and the stories that take them far and wide into worlds they hardly ever dreamed of.

It is sad when people can't find that passion. It's almost like a piece of their heart refuses to open and engage. This lack of passion can happen for all sorts of reasons but fear of letting go and surrendering to a passion probably tops the list. Fear of exposing emotions, fear of not being good enough, or even a fear of feeling too much all get in the way of finding something to be passionate about.

And now with the flood of information that we are exposed to and the wealth of entertainment that is available at the click of a button there is another reason for losing our passion. It is what they are calling "ego depletion."

In order to have passion you must hold on to a core of who you are. If that gets burnt out by too much stimulation you end up feeling drained and your passion can't get a foot hold. It is easier to curl up on a couch with the remote control for the TV.

There are people who were gourmet chefs who no longer cook, musicians who are so overwhelmed that they are no longer able to practice their instruments.

Staying motivated is fueled by passion and there are ways to stay motivated by keeping passions alive. What starts out as a natural process of engagement may have to have a boost from time to time. Getting enough rest, unplugging from all the information coming at us and simply getting away can all help in reigniting our passions.

How engaged in life would you say you are?

Julie speaks of herself

The percentage that comes to mind is 50%. I have my work and then I have my piano and the music I love. I am also engaged with my cats and care deeply about the plight of all animals on this planet. And of course I have my friends and I am very involved in these relationships that I hold dear. The rest of the time I'm on autopilot with the routines I have around my health and technology.

Olivia talks about her own blossoming

After all the Caregiving I have done in my life I am just starting to blossom now. It has taken all this time for me to get started.

I still wonder at all the Caregiving I did, all the planning and trying to get things done. It's amazing how much of my energy was given over to that.

Right now I'm living at about 65% of where I'll eventually be in terms of how engaged in my life I plan to become. When I cared for my brother I gave it 300% and that was the most engaged I've ever been in anything before or after.

Is it a comfortable level of engagement? Would you prefer to be more or less engaged?

Olivia speaks of what's comfortable for her

Right now I'm OK with where I am. I'm taking some time to get geared up. I like having a mission and I don't want to have my hands in too many pies.

Julie speaks of not being satisfied with her level of engagement in her life

No, I'm not comfortable right now. I would like to be more engaged. On some level I would like to retreat and meditate and have more time to myself. On another level I love the idea of intentional communities and that would involve more participation. There is a part of me that wants to do that in the future. I have a whole dream of shared responsibilities, getting up to go to the yoga class in the morning, taking turns making breakfast. I have an entire vision of what it would be but at the end of the day I'm still living alone in my own space.

Chapter e

Caring in faith and belief

Musings on Mayeroff:
We believe in our ability to care and we honor our need to care for others.[103]

Author's reflections:
Our ancient ancestry appears to have predisposed us to think of ourselves as a member of a tribe; in those early days it was most likely necessary for survival. We were protected by our identity with a group.
  In the modern landscape things are a bit more fluid. We have lots of choices for how we want to define our tribe and most of us take on several identities, or tribes. Men and women each have their tribal definitions, as do young and old, rich and poor. These markers allow us to gather together with others like us in a shared language and culture. In our present day, one the most obvious examples of tribes are street gangs, with their special dress and body markings, rituals and codes of conduct.
  One important way in which some humans coalesce into an identifiable tribe is through organized religion. They enjoy a feeling of belonging and safety as a member of a church. This membership sometimes can turn sour if there is a high demand for conformity in order to attain the approval and security of the group. In some cases the need to care for and express ourselves may have to be suppressed for the survival of the group. When our own ability to flourish is being threatened, there needs to be an evaluation of whether belonging to such a tribe is beneficial.

Musings on Mayeroff:
We have faith that we can learn from the experiences of our lives and that we will be attracted to a path that furthers growth the way plants in the garden turn towards the sun.[104]

Author's reflections:
Our faith in our own powers allows us to actively work on finding out what is true for us and what speaks to our heart and soul. Faith in our ability results in a life of challenge and discovery. To know what we truly believe we need to challenge, question and explore what our faith means as our life unfolds. Faith is not a static experience.
  Blind faith is a very different experience. It's like hearsay. It comes from what others have told us but isn't coming from our own life experience.

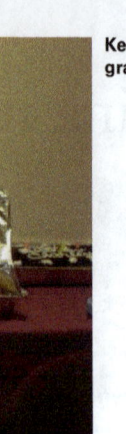

Kellie and grandpa at 85.

Do you know people who are very involved in the tenets and practices of their organized religion?

Kellie talks about her involvement in her religion

Yes, I was brought up Presbyterian. I would say that I'm faith-filled or spiritual as opposed to religious. One of the main tenets of the Presbyterian religion is pre-destination. You can choose between many paths but your final destination is pre-determined.

When you are five years old–and this is what you are told–you aren't meant to understand it. I think the bottom line is that you are going to be fine. However it ends up was how it was supposed to be all along. It is meant to be a comfort.

When I started down the long road of being a Caregiver I questioned this tenet. It caused me to more closely examine my faith. I had help from within my family. Grandpa was big in the Presbyterian church. He was an elder. My mom was an organist in the church. My dad learned the theology and almost became a minister. I was really brought up in the church and it was always present in my life.

Kellie talks about her best friend and her grandfather

My friend's husband is a Methodist minister. They are both very close to me in my life. I liked knowing that they were religious, not that we talked about it all that much, but it was more of a comfort since my whole family was involved in religion. That is, except for my stepmother who went to church but wasn't involved in religion much beyond that.

My dad was very religious and so was my Grandpa even though we didn't talk about it. Grandpa was interested in all different faiths. In going through his stuff recently, I found lots of books on the different religions. If Jehovah's Witnesses came to the door he would make them coffee and talk to them to find out what their religion was about. He would tell me that he didn't know which was the right belief. He wanted to just take it all in. In turn, I would learn about all the religions just by being there with him.

Sheri talks about the role of religion in the lives of the teachers at work

I became sort of a Caregiver for one of the other teachers at work. She teamed with me and was being abused by our principal. We all tried to protect her. The other teachers were doing prayer groups for her. They are very, very religious.

I'm the token Jewish person. They know I'm gay and are very loving and supportive. These are not issues that separates us. Their religious commitment gets them through their struggles just like my spirituality gets me through mine. My faith just isn't connected to an organized religion.

Do you discuss matters of faith with those around you?

Kellie talks about sharing her ideas about faith with others

Religion is very personal. I talk to my friend and her husband about it sometimes and I was also able to talk to my dad and Grandpa about religion when I had questions.

My religion became more important to me towards the end of Caregiving because I wanted to explore the issues and meaning of life and death. How do you have faith through all of this even when there is suffering or when things get too hard?

I started to feel that I was being selfish for forgetting that everyone suffers. My lack of generosity towards others was a reason for me to doubt my beliefs. I was trying to get a handle on things and make sense of it all in my faith. It's all a big puzzle where no one really knows the answers. It's a big question mark.

My friend's husband told me a good story. He said that God is always with us. He's like the parent that is holding our hand even when we slip and fall. He couldn't stop the fall but he's still holding our hand. I liked that image.

My dad used to talk about academic ideas in the same way, questioning, contemplating. Many of the different religions have similar ideas to each other so there are many places for me to pull my beliefs from.

Sheri talks about how she spoke about religion with her friend at work

When the principal was being difficult towards my friend I would listen to my friend's side and consider the source of what was being said about her. Religion is often about comfort, and because religion was important for my friend, I would say, "I'll hold you in my prayers," or, "Remember that God is in charge." I wanted to show that I supported her in a language that she could relate to.

How thoughtful are the people in your life about their religion?

Kellie talks about her ex-husband's struggles with his religion

My dad, granddad, best friend and her husband are all very thoughtful and could discuss ideas of faith. My ex-husband is very black and white. He was brought up Catholic and is very religious in his own way. He goes back and forth with the church. I'm not Catholic and was married before. He was mad at his religion because we couldn't get married in the church because of my divorce. There was a lot of his questioning his faith and how they could do that and not take into account our situation.

I didn't talk about religion with him because it brought up a lot of emotion as it is so personal for him. If he brought it up occasionally we'd talk about it. He's been in a constant struggle with the Catholic Church, however I don't think he would ever convert to anything else.

Sheri talks about how much the teachers at work think about their religion

My co-workers at school are very connected to their religion and think about it a lot. Their religion guides them to care about others. As a result I experience their care when I'm at work. I really found a family there and missing them is the hardest part of not working right now. They are still reaching out to me.

Are others curious about your beliefs?

Kellie talks about her friends' curiosity about her religion

Yes, my friends and I can talk about everything. I find that my friends and co-workers are especially curious about the structure of the Presbyterian Church. Our church has a lot of committees and government is the model for the organization.

Sheri talks about the teachers at work being curious about her religion

One person and her husband asked me about my beliefs. They were asking why I don't believe in Jesus the same way they do. They were younger, in their thirties, and really didn't know the differences in our religions. They weren't pushing the idea of conversion.

After we had our conversation, when it was her turn to lead the daily prayer she would now say "in God's name" instead, of "in Jesus's name." The other teachers are older and already know about Judaism, but in some ways they were less sensitive to my beliefs. They have asked about foods for Chanukah and one gave me a Chanukah gift. It doesn't bother me which name you use in prayers because I just feel they are different names for similar concepts we have about God.

In the Jewish religion we aren't supposed to spell out the word God so we use G-D. Some of the teachers understood this and would explain it to the others. I end up doing it their way sometimes and spelling the whole word out.

How does their faith comfort them?

Kellie wasn't able to find out how her dad's faith comforted him before he died

I didn't talk about what my father's beliefs were about dying because he tended towards depression and I was afraid to bring it up. I also didn't expect him to die when he did so there wasn't time to discuss or prepare for his death. All he said was that he wanted to be cremated.

Kellie talks about her step-mother's conflict with her faith

I was able to talk to my step-mother about her impending death. She had stage four cancer so she knew how it all would end. She was at peace with her death but had many struggles with God. Part of this was because her son was very against the concept of God because he couldn't understand how God could let good people suffer.

Sheri talks about how faith comforts the teachers at work

I think for the teachers at work their religion gives them the strength to get through the day when they are having difficulties. Not only that but when they are uncertain or afraid, their religion comforts them. One of their husbands has been out of work and this couple's faith helps them deal with it. We all believe that in the timing of how things unfold, he'll get the best job. That's faith. Right now his grandmother got hurt and now that he's out of work he's her Caregiver. He's done it before so it's a good match and the timing was perfect. It's a feeling that God is blessing us, because he is now available to help her.

When you really believe in the best sense of the word there is security in that and comfort. There's the trust and faith in the unknown.

Does your caring affect your faith or vice versa?

Kellie talks generally about those she cared for

I was influenced by the faith of each person I was caring for in how I approached them. When my step-mother got sick my father needed comfort.

He didn't deal well with anything negative, so when she found out she had cancer he had trouble dealing with it. As I talked more to him about his faith during these tough times, then my faith actually got stronger.

Near my stepmother's death I was taking care of her and my dad. As my faith was getting stronger my step-brother's faith was getting weaker. He would doubt God and ask why all the bad things were happening. My step-brother took everything a different way. He could only see the suffering but not the love in the situation. His struggle with his faith didn't affect mine. I just realized that I saw everything very differently.

As everyone was getting sick my grandfather was internalizing everything, which wasn't good for him but at least I was spared his emotions. I was too young at the time to realize that he was having problems and as a child didn't need to be exposed to that much struggle in the adults around me. I had already lost my mother through divorce.

Kellie talks about the effect of her stepmother's faith on her

My stepmother's faith was absent in her life. She would go to church, but her faith wasn't in the forefront like it was in my father's life. Even though her faith was weak, mine got stronger during the time I cared for her. It must have been because of the conversations I was having with my dad about what it means to be human in this world and our spirituality beyond that. It became bigger than just religion for me. I still say my prayers at night but it takes on a shape that permeates my life.

The Presbyterian idea of predestination fits in with my values and how I live my life. I've known from an early age that there will be a good ending and I chose the path I want to walk to get there. They believe that you will receive the grace that you were born with in the end. It could come earlier if you are a very spiritual person and become enlightened during your lifetime.

The idea is that even if you are experiencing something bad it will eventually work itself out. It's like the play Annie with the song "Tomorrow". Have faith in this and just keep going is the message.

That's what I got out of taking care of my stepmother.

Kellie talks about the effects of her dad's death on her faith

When my father died, it was a real shock. Multiple Sclerosis isn't supposed to kill you and he could have lived into his 80's. In terms of my faith I didn't lose my beliefs when he died because I think his beliefs fortified mine. He seemed to have died because he loved his second wife so much that he just couldn't live without her after she died of cancer. There's something very profound and loving about that. She was the strong one and he wasn't.

That's why my parents originally got divorced. They were too similar. They both needed someone to lean on and when they tried with each other they both fell down. My stepmother was strong for my dad. He had needed someone stronger and that was true in death as well. He died a short while after my stepmom.

Sheri talks about her faith coming before her caring

If I'm more balanced because of my spirituality then I feel that I'm more aligned with the universe and that is my faith. However, I don't need to give to someone to feel close to God. I look at it that God is coming through me as I give to others. I feel that God loves me no matter what I do.

Author's reflections:
Fear is a powerful force and is almost the opposite of faith. Rulers have used fear to keep their populations submissive. Advertisers have used it to sell everything from home security systems to tooth paste.

Fear can also be self-perpetuating. The more we fear life the more we close ourselves off to life. The unknown future becomes an excuse to contract. We create in our minds a worst-case scenario for the future.

In this fearful state we are no longer concerned with our emotional, spiritual or artistic growth or the growth of others. Security and survival become our only focus.

Musings on Mayeroff:
Trust and confidence accompany faith as we travel into an unknowable future of our caring for another and growing through our caring.[105]

Author's reflections:
When we have faith and have adjusted to the fact that we can't know the future before it happens, we can let go of trying to "push the river." In our Caregiving we often don't know what health, financial or emotional issues are around the bend. When we trust that somehow in our caring we'll get through it and grow from our experiences, we gain the confidence that flows from living in this caring way.

Do you have trust and confidence in your path even though the outcome may be unknown?

Kellie talks about her periodic doubts

I don't always have trust or confidence that I have chosen the right path. Since I am Presbyterian they say the outcome is set. It's like individual battles in a war may have different outcomes, but the overall outcome is known according to my religion.

Sometimes I doubt for five minutes and sometimes it's a day. After my father and stepmother died I probably had a couple of months of doubt. It's scary when everything is thrown at you like that and you just don't know what to do. You get through everything you are supposed to do on autopilot and about six months later you just stop. I finally realized I had just lost half of my family. It's tough.

My age probably played into it as well. Young people go to war and don't worry about death. Now that I'm older, I can be more retrospective.

Sheri talks about trusting her path

I would say mostly yes that I have trust in my path. It doesn't mean that fear doesn't sometimes creep in. Because of my faith the majority of the time the answer is yes I trust my path. I feel that there are no other choices in this that will still bring me joy.

Chapter f

Caring as gratitude

Musings on Mayeroff:
Caring for others fills us with gratitude as does giving to others: as we care and give we get to grow and live the meaning in our lives and this is what we become especially grateful for.

Life is full of surprises and these twists and turns along the road of our lives give us the opportunity to react to people and situations outside of our conscious control. We appreciate that we are dependent on many things that we can't control and our willing dependency on this serendipity liberates us from having to control every aspect of our lives.

In the end we finally realize that the truth is that we have received many unexpected gifts and surprises during our lives that we would never have thought to ask for and that we were lucky to be blessed with.[106]

Author's reflections:
It has been scientifically proved that the feeling of gratitude makes us happy. In Martin Seligman's book "Authentic Happiness" he adds the feelings of satisfaction to gratitude, naming it gratification, as more a cause for true happiness than either alone.

As seen through the lens of gratitude and satisfaction, Caregiving takes on an entirely new perspective. Helping others now becomes a gift because we realize that through our Caregiving we are also given the ability to learn about ourselves and to grow during the experience. This fills our hearts with gratitude and satisfaction for a life well lived.

Dependency on surprise, chance, and serendipity relieves us of the notion that we are in control of every aspect of our challenges. This view of dependency, that Meyeroff speaks of, takes on a new perspective for us when we accept it in gratitude. It becomes a gift to be grateful for. As we surrender the impossible feeling of total control we can relax into other dependencies: on people, on institutions, on help with a sense of gratitude for what is being offered and our ability to accept these gifts.

How do you generally feel about dependency? What happens in dependency? What are the positive and negative aspects of dependency in Caregiving?

Christie talks about her husband's growing dependency

Since I had decided not to have children I had never experienced that kind of total dependency. I thought I would have trouble as I cared for my husband with his dependency on me. I enjoy my independence and liked the independent style of relationship that my husband and I had enjoyed for over twenty years. We pursued our separate interests and then came together for the things we liked to share.

I had never allowed myself to be needed much or to be needy with my friends for much more than my friendship, companionship and shared interests. We liked our independence but we were still young and able.

I suppose my growing interest in sharing my life with the avian species was getting me ready for what was to come with my husband. Compared to cats or dogs, birds as companions are low maintenance. Food, warmth, interaction and a place to sleep at night were all those little parakeets needed. These were my baby steps towards starting to be needed.

Once my husband started down the road of dementia I slowly realized he would be dependent on me to varying degrees for many years to come. Maybe due to the fact that it was a gradual process I willingly took on each new level of dependency as it came. I think I secretly thought of the challenges as problems that needed solving and didn't think of how much I was now needed as compared to before.

The darker side of Caregiving was seeing that I am not an endless stream of generosity and love. I can get burnt out and there was much to learn that I didn't take advantage of during my Caregiving years. My wanting to be strong, in control and independent in my Caregiving actually impeded my ability to find resources that would have lightened my load during the eight years that I cared for my husband.

At the time I didn't see the truth that my being dependent on the course of my husband's illness ultimately got me to give up control. Once I gave up trying to control the situation I was finally able to focus on learning what was needed and got the help that had been available all along. It was liberating and I carry these lessons with me.

Joe P. talks about mutual dependency with his friend

My friend and I are Caregivers for each other. When there's a mutual Caregiving and you feel there is a balance, there is the beautiful exchange of energy. It is a light and joyous dependency. We are able to take turns without pressure because next week it will be my turn.

Usually I think of the word dependency as a heavy and limiting thing. I think it can confine you both intellectually and emotionally. I am actually finding that as I allow myself to become dependent on another person, like my friend, I begin to appreciate his gifts, what he has to give, and I sometimes sit there in utter amazement. It is truly something that I am grateful for.

I see his strengths, like how intellectual he is and how deep his emotions run. I end up loving him more as I experience his capabilities. If I had not

Chris F. and Joe P.

allowed myself to be dependent on him I would never have discovered these things about him. He feels the same way about being dependent on me. There is a constant dialogue between us.

It is important that we can share our weaknesses without feeling like the other person will attack. As he shares with me his weakness about his struggle with food and overeating, I treat him like the intellectual that he is and we look for solutions to his issues. I also understand that this issue has nothing to do with intelligence. He has an emotional problem when it comes to controlling his food intake. I try to be supportive without attacking or being condescending. This is an example of the trust we have with each other.

Musings on Mayeroff:
Until we have actually expressed our appreciation to others and thanked them, our gratitude remains incomplete, inside us. By caring for others we show our appreciation for what we have received throughout our life. When we connect our caring to our gratitude it makes it easier to care even more.[107]

Author's reflections:
Life Coaches are taught to acknowledge clients for their efforts, to express appreciation for their accomplishments and to be sure to celebrate with them when they reach their goals. These are the central tenets of the profession. It is not enough to create a plan, execute the plan and find success. Having someone there to appreciate your hard work and perseverance is just as important in order to experience a happy, fulfilling life. It is also way more fun to celebrate with someone who has your best interests at heart. To celebrate as a lonely party of one brings us nowhere near the joy when we share our moments of exhilaration and accomplishment with others.

Keeping our appreciation to ourselves for the things and people we are grateful for is like going to a baseball game gagged. Letting people know what they mean to us and how much we are grateful for their place in our life is as important as telling them that we love them.

One way to show that appreciation is to care for them when they need us. This becomes our expression of the appreciation for the gifts they have given us throughout our earlier lives together. This can spiral into caring more deeply for them now as we connect it to our gratitude for what they truly mean and have meant to us.

Is it easy for you to express appreciation? What have you noticed when you were able to tell someone how much they helped you? What stops you from telling someone how much you appreciate them?

Christie talks about showing appreciation to her new boyfriend

My boyfriend and I originally met a few years after I got together with my husband. We hit it off right away as friends. We were both competitive athletes and had many interests in common. I became his massage therapist and later his acupuncturist and we stayed friends over the years. He became my weightlifting coach and took me all the way to world level competition. His wife died in the late 90's, and shortly after that my husband started showing signs of dementia.

We lost contact towards the end of my husband's illness. I had too much on my plate and he was keeping his life on track. We united again for the Thanksgiving weekend the year after my husband died and rekindled our friendship, only this time it has grown into more. We have joined as life partners for the past four years and our love continues to grow.

He is a generous man and often it is hard for me to find the words to express my appreciation. He has helped me with my finances and supports every project I take on. Since the words are difficult for me, I try to express my appreciation in other ways. I'm supportive of his projects and welcome him into all aspects of my life.

Sometimes I think it is just a matter of getting used to being involved with someone who prefers a more active participation in each other's life. My husband had been more distant in that way. I also wonder about whether I have any leftover fears that this kind of close relationship is a reminder of the deeper involvement that came with my husband's illness. I think it will be a matter of time and trust for me to be able to show my appreciation more freely.

Joe P. talks about appreciating his mentor to his son

When I talk to my mentor's son it is easy to tell him how much his dad meant to me and how having him in my life was an amazing experience for me. I will never forget the gift of our relationship and it still influences me.

It makes him very happy to have these new insights into his father and to hear things about him that he never knew. It gives him a greater understanding of who his father was and helps him feel closer to him.

In other situations generally speaking I'm afraid of showing my appreciation because of the depth of feeling I have for a person. I'm afraid that the other person wouldn't be able to accept the level of my appreciation which sometimes feels like a force of nature.

Musings on Mayeroff:
Much of existence can't be known, but in our lives there is room to explore and connect with others. In our exploration we often sense a deep order to our lives that goes beyond our limited human comprehension. We are left without words to describe what we sense intuitively. This sense of order and connection gives us a way to find our joy.

As we live our lives independently we are happy for the connections that bring us together with others. Our gratitude comes with the joy of experiencing sharing. We owe our joy to these connections.[108]

Author's reflections:
All over the world, in almost all cultures, you can find strong bonds between individuals and their community. Hunters go out and bring back food to share with their tribe. Gatherers bring back vegetation and herbs to nourish and heal others. These are connections that have traditionally held groups together. We bond to each other in a very natural way. In addition we have the experience of communal joy, music and celebration that connects us. We can be grateful to these connections for our very survival.

The mysteries of our lives are shared in communal stories, dreams and mythology. These myths cross over from culture to culture and highlight the order we discover in our lives. They help to cement the connections that we have to each other. Life seems to also make sense in some very fundamental way beyond words. Again, we can be glad for these ways to connect to our communities.

Does your life seem to have a deep order when you look back over your life?

Christie talks about her life making sense

I remember Joseph Campbell talking to Bill Moyers just before his death. In his 80's, he said as looked back over his life that everything seemed to fit and make sense.

As much as I would prefer to take away the memories of any suffering

I have endured or any sadness or confusion I have experienced, I have an equally strong belief that I am like a picture puzzle and all the pieces of my life have been needed to create the whole.

Caring for my husband was probably the biggest emotional growth spurt I could ever have experienced. That's why I cringe when people talk about Alzheimer's as only a tragedy. There is so much to be grateful for in caring for someone with this disease. Without this experience I wouldn't be where I am today. At the age of 60 I already have the feeling that what Joseph Campbell was referring to has been true in my life as well. Things do seem to make sense over a life time. This doesn't take away from the feeling that I have much yet to create and discover.

Joe P. talks about his life as he looks back

Yes, there is a thread that runs all through my life. The theme is the wisdom and greater understanding of humanity I gained as a result of always caring for others. My whole life is about being able to walk a mile in another's shoes and I am grateful that I have always had an uncanny ability to commiserate with my fellow human beings.

Who are our hero Caregivers?

Alicia moved to Puerto Rico during her mother's last three months before she died of cancer. Her dad is still alive and she cares for him long distance as he gets older and more frail. She also cares for her Yoga students in individual sessions or group classes.

Barb cared for her father from a distance who was living with an aneurysm. Her mother was the primary Caregiver. Once he died Barb has continued to care for her mother who is now in her nineties, still works and has an active life in Florida. Recently her mother has been experiencing many medical issues and Barb's Caregiving has stepped up its pace. Barb frequently travels to Florida to help get her mother the best medical care available. Her brother is also involved in the Caregiving for their mom.

Barbara, the mother of two teenagers, cared for her husband during his cancer. She now guides other Caregivers as they journey down a similar road.

Chris F. helped his mother as she took care of his father for 2 ½ years when he started having signs of dementia. His father had been a minister and a very powerful person in the community. His mother didn't understand Alzheimer's disease and didn't have the skills to adapt as her husband declined. Her lack of skills for dealing with her husband was frustrating for him to be around. Chris lived with his parents at the time and only found respite at work. He also took care of his mother when she became ill and now he cares for his sister. She has mental illness and lives with him in their family home. He is also a union representative and cares deeply about his job and his union members. He has also been involved with caring for an ex-fiancee and still cares deeply for her family.

Christie took care of her husband for eight years as he lived with early onset Alzheimer's disease. She kept him at home for seven years with very little support from the outside world. Her entire family is on the west coast and she lives in New York.
    She had also cared for her Grandmother both when she broke her hip and then during the last three years that she suffered with colon cancer.
Her father, her grandfather, and her sister's mother-in-law also had dementia towards the end of their lives and her mother, grandmother and sister respectively were their Caregivers. Christie comes from a family of Caregivers.

Claudine cared for both her parents before they died. They were living in other states and Canada during that time so she would travel to them when she could. She also cares for her husband who is a diabetic. Her daughter was recently diagnosed with an autoimmune disease that the doctors are still looking into. When her brother-in-law had a car accident and was confined to a wheel chair, she and her husband would travel an hour each way to give his sister a break from her Caregiving.

Debbie cared for her mother before she died. She took care of the finances and visited as much as she could. She had two sisters who helped. One lived near their mom and did the primary Caregiving and the other was a nurse and helped with the medical issues. The three sisters were able to guide their mother from the brink of financial ruin. They moved her from a house that was in foreclosure into a rental home in the town where they grew up.

Debbie also is caring from a distance for her husband's aunt who has Alzheimer's. She and her husband offer telephone support to her brother-in-law and and his wife who are the primary caregivers and visit when they can.

Joe M. is a retired business owner. He cared for his wife when she was diagnosed with cancer until she died. His kids are very close to him and he is slowly getting back to a more active social life.

Joe P. was a long-term, long distance Caregiver for his frail, elderly father. He would go to visit whenever he could. At an earlier time he had already helped his father for eleven years to care for his mother who eventually died of Alzheimer's.

After his mother died he had cared for his own wife during the three months before she died from cancer. After caring for his father he later took care of his friend and mentor who became more frail as he was dying of cancer.

He has many other friends and cares for them in different ways, including being a mentor for them. They return the caring when they can. There is one special young man that Joe P. cared for in his teens whose parents were unavailable due to their work. This young friend would spend summers and holidays with Joe and his wife. They lost track of each other for ten years and only recently have reconnected and their bond is even stronger than before. He also has another great friend from his martial arts training and the caring is equal and deep on both sides. They are very involved in each other's daily lives and support each other in a variety of ways.

Julie cared for her father and then extensively for her mother before she died. She has also cared for a friend with mental illness and another friend as he experienced severe medical problems.

Keith has two adopted sons. One is on the autism spectrum and one has dyslexia. Beyond being their parent he has been handling all the issues that have come up for them over the years in school and sports. They are both in their early twenties and they are now both addicted to drugs and alcohol. Keith's wife does the bulk of the logistical Caregiving while he is at work. He supports her emotionally by allowing her to vent whenever she needs to and he has given the boys jobs and a home until they can work things out. He is also caring for his mom who is able to stay in her home with the help of 24 hour care. He also helped his wife take care of her mother and is now helping her care for the woman who took care of both of their moms. She has had cancer and has no family or resources. They help with rent and getting her to appointments.

Kellie from the age of ten cared for her father who was diagnosed with Multiple Sclerosis. While her father was still alive she then cared for her step mother who was diagnosed with cancer. After they both died within a month of each other she lived with her grandfather until she got married. When he had his stroke she arranged for his care and he lived until this past year. She is experiencing herself for the first time in years without her Caregiving responsibilities.

Liz cared for her mother-in-law both while she briefly moved in with her family and then later when she went to live in a facility. Her mother-in-law not only had Alzheimer's but was also addicted to narcotic pain killers. Liz was raising her young children at home at the time and had the flexibility of an open schedule so she could be available. Her husband came from a large family and Liz had to negotiate her care through his family's wishes.

She is also caring for her mother who has Rheumatoid Arthritis and is aging. When her dad had dementia, she cared for him and her mom whenever she was needed. The rest of the family was out of town so it fell on her. At the same time she has been raising her two daughters who are now in their early twenties.

Her husband has had prostate cancer and she helped him adjust emotionally as he recovered after his surgery.

Marian cared for her husband for 6 years before he died. He had dementia and diabetes. He died at the age of 92 and was quite frail in the end. She insisted on keeping him in their home and brought in hospice to help with the end stages of his life. She has four daughters, three of which are spread out all over the country. The youngest is nearby and they are very close. She has 7 grandchildren and two great grandchildren. Her oldest daughter, the author of this book, was caring for her own husband with early onset Alzheimer's disease and they shared a similar path. Both husbands died within six months of each other.

Earlier in her life she took care of her own father when her mother could no longer handle the situation. He was in the later stages of Alzheimer's and she was able to place him in a facility near her home until he died. Her four daughters were young at the time and there was no way to have her father move in with them.

Olivia took care of her ex-boyfriend who was a Veteran and had PTSD for 6 or 7 years. In addition she cared for her sick brother who was also a veteran, a drug addict and eventually died of HIV. He had been living with their mother who eventually started showing signs of dementia. Olivia cared for both of them when they lived together and then she cared for her mother who was in a nursing home for the last ten years of her life with dementia. Her brother was also institutionalized because he needed custodial care.

A much older brother who was Schizophrenic had been institutionalized for as long as Olivia could remember and she cared for him once her parents were no longer able to. As he aged he became a senior with other health problems and due to his mental illness was in and out of many nursing homes before he died.

Patrice cares for her son who has autism. She is a full time writer and writes a column about family life on the autistic spectrum. She has three children 13, 10 and 8. She lost her first baby six months into the pregnancy. Her goal is to share her experiences with other parents walking a similar path with their children through the autistic spectrum experience so that they can feel connected to her and each other. She is also an Associate with the Sisters of Charity of New York. They base their work on that of Saint Elizabeth Seton who was also a mother and wife and inspires Patrice in her Caregiving.

Sarah cared for her mother during her cancer. They hadn't gotten along very well before but Sarah felt she needed to do this for her widowed mother, especially in the face of their previous relationship. She felt proud that she was able to rise up to the challenge and be a caring person when it was most important. Now she is also the facilitator of a support group of partners and spouses of people who have cancer. While she was facilitating this group her life partner was diagnosed with cancer and she became a Caregiver again.

Sheri was a teacher who cared deeply for her students and colleagues. She was also a Caregiver for a neighbor who had problems with drug addiction and eventually committed suicide. In her relationship with her partner there were several examples of caring that came to mind, reminding us that caring and Caregiving have a lot of emotional overlaps.

Susan is taking care of her husband who has early-onset Alzheimer's disease. She also has her two young grandchildren living with them. She has a good friend who shares in some of the caring for her husband.

Suzanne took care of her husband for many years after his kidneys were destroyed in a surgery to remove stones. She became more involved once he had the two kidney transplants. The last five months of his life were the most intense part of her Caregiving. She had her daughter's support throughout. They were doing very technical medical procedures at home so that he could stay home as much as possible. Earlier in his life he had had Crohn's disease but he handled all that himself.

Terry cared for her father who eventually died of cancer while in hospice care. She was joined by her brother, her sister and her mother in the Caregiving. They all had jobs but she organized the care. She has a very demanding job and was able to keep up her duties because she had the rest of her family's support. Her brother has cancer, but she has decided to focus on caring for her mother as she adjusts to life now without her husband. She is also a long distance Caregiver for her great aunt in Florida.

Toni took care of her mother many years ago when she developed Early Onset Alzheimer's. This was way before most people knew anything about the disease. Her father was still alive at the time and they worked as a team to care for her mother. Probably due to the stress, he died before his wife. Her brother has had a rare health condition and she has cared for him by travelling to his city every weekend and giving him moral support when he would get discouraged. He is mostly recovered now. She teaches young children and cares for them and the other teachers she works with. They have become a family. She also cared for a neighbor who was addicted to drugs and finally committed suicide. She is in a deeply caring relationship with her partner.

About the Author

As a director can direct themselves in a movie, I have two roles in When the Voiceless Sing, author and Caregiver. I've reflected on what each topic presented and answered the questions in several sections as Christie. Being a participant in the process gave me a chance to review my role as Caregiver for my husband and share my story. As the author I have been able to organize the information and have it flow from topic to topic. Both experiences have been rewarding and helped so much in my growth as a person.

After writing my memoir **Living on the Verge of Insanity** in 2007 I have worked with hundreds of Caregivers in my local community. I have often been privileged to hear their very emotional stories. In this book I've worked to give a flavor of what Caregivers have in common as well as what makes them different from each other. No story is exactly alike but every story fits into what it means to be a Caregiver.

My next project is to train Professional Caregiver Advocates (PCA) to sit with families as they struggle to find their own answers. Each PCA will become the activist in their community to rally around programs and resources that will benefit their local Caregiving community. By the time you've read this book we shall be well on our way towards realizing this dream of helping to make life a little easier for each and every Caregiver.

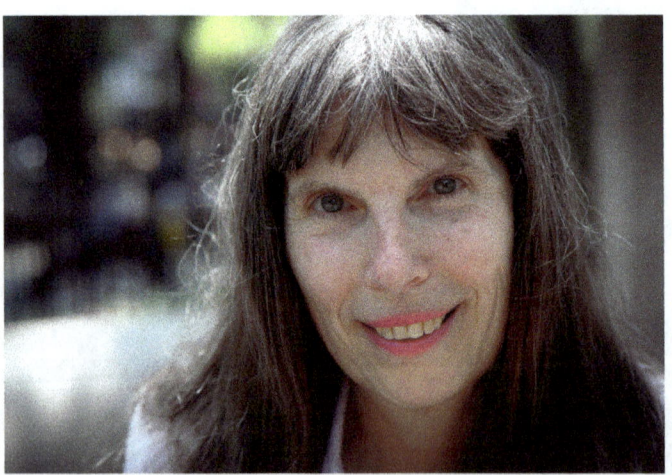

Resources

Visit www.caregiveraccess.org
Caregiver Access is free and easy to use with everything in one place:
- suggested questions to ask related to Caregiving
- glossaries of technical terms
- directory of contacts - professionals waiting to help
- free programs for Caregivers including support groups and coaching
- conditions – links to what national organizations are doing for families and Caregivers
- Caregiver stories – you are not alone!

www.caregiveraccess.blogspot.com
News, articles and links for Family and Informal Caregivers

www.livingontheverge.com
Living on the Verge of Insanity is Christine Sotmary's first book, a memoir of her Caregiving experience.

https://www.facebook.com/#!/groups/171473826255114/
Post articles, photos, stories and videos related to your Caregiving

http://whenthevoicelesssing.blogspot.com/
Additional stories from the Caregivers in the book.

End Notes

1. Milton Mayeroff, On Caring (Perennial Library: Harper & Row, 1971) 5
2. Mayeroff 7
3. Mayeroff 11
4. Mayeroff 10
5. Mayeroff 5 – 6
6. Mayeroff 11
7. Mayeroff 8
8. Mayeroff 8
9. Mayeroff 8 – 9
10. Mayeroff 9
11. Mayeroff 9
12. Mayeroff 8
13. Mayeroff 13
14. Mayeroff 13
15. Mayeroff 14
16. Mayeroff 13
17. Mayeroff 15 – 16
18. Mayeroff 16
19. Mayeroff 16
20. Mayeroff 16
21. Mayeroff 17
22. Mayeroff 18
23. Mayeroff 18
24. Mayeroff 19
25. Mayeroff 19
26. Mayeroff 19
27. Mayeroff 20
28. Mayeroff 19
29. Mayeroff 20 – 21
30. Mayeroff 22
31. Mayeroff 22
32. Mayeroff 23 – 24
33. Mayeroff 25
34. Mayeroff 24
35. Mayeroff 23
36. Mayeroff 25
37. Mayeroff 25
38. Mayeroff 25
39. Mayeroff 25 – 26
40. Mayeroff 26 – 27
41. Mayeroff 27
42. Mayeroff 27 – 28
43. Mayeroff 27
44. Mayeroff 30
45. Mayeroff 29 – 30
46. Mayeroff 29 – 30
47. Mayeroff 30
48. Mayeroff 31
49. Mayeroff 33
50. Mayeroff 33
51. Mayeroff 34
52. Mayeroff 35
53. Mayeroff 35
54. Mayeroff 35 - 36
55. Mayeroff 36 – 37
56. Mayeroff 37 – 38
57. Mayeroff 37
58. Mayeroff 38
59. Mayeroff 38
60. Mayeroff 41 – 42
61. Mayeroff 43
62. Mayeroff 43
63. Mayeroff 44
64. Mayeroff 44
65. Mayeroff 48
66. Mayeroff 48
67. Mayeroff 48
68. Mayeroff 51
69. Mayeroff 52
70. Mayeroff 52
71. Mayeroff 53
72. Mayeroff 54
73. Mayeroff 57
74. Mayeroff 54 - 55
75. Mayeroff 54
76. Mayeroff 57
77. Mayeroff 56
78. Mayeroff 56
79. Mayeroff 59
80. Mayeroff 59
81. Mayeroff 61
82. Mayeroff 64
83. Mayeroff 65
84. Mayeroff 69 - 70
85. Mayeroff 67
86. Mayeroff 70
87. Mayeroff 73 - 74
88. Mayeroff 73
89. Mayeroff 74
90. Mayeroff 74
91. Mayeroff 75
92. Mayeroff 76
93. Mayeroff 77
94. Mayeroff 77
95. Mayeroff 77
96. Mayeroff 77 - 78
97. Mayeroff 78
98. Mayeroff 80
99. Mayeroff 80
100. Mayeroff 80
101. Mayeroff 81 - 82
102. Mayeroff 82
103. Mayeroff 83
104. Mayeroff 83
105. Mayeroff 84
106. Mayeroff 85 - 86
107. Mayeroff 86
108. Mayeroff 86

Index of Caregivers

Alicia - chapters 15, 22,
Barb - chapters 21, a
Barbara - chapters 8, 16, 26
Chris F. - chapters 5, 14
Christie - chapters 4, 7, 11, 17, 23, 25, 27, a, f
Claudine - chapters 17, 24, c
Debbie - chapters 1, 3, 24
Joe M. - chapters 10, 19, 27
Joe P. - chapters 2, 4, 19, f
Julie - chapters 25, d
Keith - chapters 6, b,
Kellie - chapters 1, 3, e
Liz - chapters 6, 12, 18
Marian - chapters 13, 18, c
Olivia - chapters 26, d
Patrice - chapters 10, 13,
Sarah - chapters 7, 11, 14, 20
Sheri - chapters 7, 22, e,
Susan - chapters 5, 8, 16
Suzanne - chapters 9, 12, 20
Terry - chapters 2, 15, 23
Toni - chapters 9, 21, b

Caregiver Notes:

Caregiver Notes:

Order Form

Copy and send order form to:
When the Voiceless Sing
c/o Christine Sotmary
P.O. Box 513
Crompond, NY 10517
USA

Item ID: WVS 1st edition
Description: When The Voiceless Sing: Love stories from our hero Caregivers
Unit Price: $24.95
Quantity:
Amount Subtotal:
Tax 8.5%:
Shipping & Handling (per book): $3.00

Total:
Currency is in U.S. Dollars (USD).

Please make check payable to: **Caregiver Access**

Shipping Info:

Name _____

Address _____

City _____ State _____ Zip _____

Country _____

Telephone _____

Email _____

www.ingramcontent.com/pod-product-compliance
Lightning Source LLC
Chambersburg PA
CBHW071700160426
43195CB00012B/1535